Madness at Midnight

I0099910

By Bianca Benjamin

"One million people commit suicide every year"
World Health Organisation

Published by:
Chipmukapublishing
PO Box 6872
Brentwood
Essex
CM13 1ZT
United Kingdom

www.chipmunkapublishing.com

Copyright © 2006 Bianca Benjamin

ISBN 978-1-905610-49-5

Acknowledgments

I dedicate this book to those patients of both Chase Farm and Charing Cross Hospitals for their unstinting support throughout difficult years. I applaud their courage and strength. Then my thanks go to Gillian and Simon Enthoven who have typed this manuscript despite my execrable handwriting. Their dedication is deeply appreciated.

Foreword

We are obsessed by the 'occult', the hidden forces of nature and the Universe. Consider all the movies and stories from Stephen King to the Blair Witch Project to the Omen series of horror movies - the unknown and inexplicable holds us in its thrall. Here is a story of an actual encounter with deep dark and largely inexplicable forces. Not a nice comfortable story with a nice fancy ending but a raw, blasting story of trials and challenges that most of us are fortunate enough not to experience and not to encounter.

Many who purport to be religious teachers teach, in the main, that the occult is dangerous and to be avoided. But this is impossible as it is all around us, it is the hidden and subtle forces of the Universe and we choose not to hear them and attempt to understand them at our peril. The battle of light and dark forces goes on in the manifest cosmos and we experience the effects both in the external arena of everyday life and in the internal arena of our inner world, our dreams and our impulses. Bianca's story shows that the hidden forces affect life and can open us up to a wider reality which is tough, challenging and dangerous. I would add that the only thing more dangerous is ignorance, and pretence that its not there. Preparation is all. To engage in battle with the subtle forces of yourself and life, inner healing is needed, healing of the wounds of childhood especially is required to help one balance one's personality and become well grounded to deal with multi-dimensional reality.

As Carlos Castaneda has written about and many shamans and spiritual teachers teach, and as corroborated by modern day quantum physicists, the reality we perceive is made up of what can best be classified as vibrations. We each of us are an Energy Body within which is the physical body.

Within the Energy Body is a point the shamans call the Assemblage Point. Which of the multitude of vibrations available we experience as 'reality' depends on the position of the Assemblage Point within our Energy Body. Move this point and the reality we perceive changes. All spiritual disciplines have at their root methods to shift the Assemblage Point in small gradual increments which we can handle and which help us gradually to learn to manoeuvre in wider realities. Bianca experienced massive sudden shifts and the results were traumatic and excruciatingly difficult.

Some years ago at a Transpersonal Psychology conference I heard first hand the story of an 'alien abductee'. As I listened most carefully to his story of abduction by aliens, in my mind I heard a shamanic journey. It felt to me like a deep visionary inner journey which took place in parallel reality, the one that can be so easily dismissed as 'imagination'. He was convinced it happened in this third dimensional everyday reality. At times in life it can be very difficult to be certain just which reality one is in. Indeed just what reality is.

The story that follows is a dramatic reminder that the world around us, which we so easily take for granted, is actually nothing more than a perception and is only as stable as the position of our Assemblage Point. Many who are considered crazy are actually perceiving realities closed to the majority of people and which conventional 'wisdom' asserts do not exist. Modern psychiatric drugs dull the senses, cut off perception and suppress the emotions thus apparently stabilizing the sufferer. But at a substantial price. The price of deadness, dulled sensibilities, lack of feelings. There must be another way and perhaps this harrowing story will help open up dialogue about the perception of wider realities and what is real in a much wider framework than presently accepted, and also just what 'mental illness' really is and when it is not illness at all but the ability to perceive a much wider band of vibrations than that normally open to the majority of people.

Leo Rutherford

Chapter One
Metapsychosis: A Journey into Schizophrenia

I've told everyone, family and friends, that I'm writing a book on my mental illness. So I guess I'd better start it. This despite the fact that I have no inspiration, no input from the subconscious mind to the conscious, no motivation. This account will be written from conscious will. Right now I have no motivation, and the simplest tasks are complicated. It's an effort to do the washing up or put my clothes in the washing machine. I am also agoraphobic which means that leaving my flat is a problem. At one stage this was so aggravated that I hired minicabs to do my shopping I have few friends. Care in the community is a joke. The community has nothing in common with the mentally ill, and the latter have nothing in common with the community. It's a catch 22 condition for in fact my closest friends right now are both mentally ill and yet I long to be in harmony with those who are well and whole. Yet I feel a sense of alienation when I am with those who are well. The precise nature of my illness is mysterious. I have labelled myself a schizophrenic in line with the diagnosis given me by the Schizophrenic Fellowship. However psychiatrists have been at a loss to diagnose my illness. The Charing Cross Hospital has stated that I'm a manic depressive. Chase Farm Hospital have found my illness puzzling and have been reluctant to put a name on it. I wish to say that the illness is painful and gives rise to thoughts of suicide. How did it all start, for I became mentally ill rather late in life at the age of fifty-two. The roots may go back to genetics to which partially I have no access. My father's line is known and carries no mental illness. My mother was adopted and her line is unknown. But from my personal point of view the whole story began in Montreal in 1980.

At that time I was married to my second husband Kwabena a neurophysiologist who was on a year's exchange to the

9

Medical School at Montreal University. Our marriage was on the rocks - he was nineteen years younger than myself and our personalities were incompatible. The only thing that bound us was sex. I had left my twin boys behind in England. Adrian was left with a friend Vera Matoorah and Leon was in boarding school at Bembridge in the Isle of Wight. He was left under the custody of my friend Alan Goodwin, a homosexual living in Hackney. Unfortunately Leon chose not to spend his holidays with Alan, so jetted back and forth between friends. I became pregnant by Kwabena in October 1980. Our marriage was virtually over but Kwabena was delighted that I was to bear his child. I had recently met with a Christian group of reborn Christians and felt that after many years of agnosticism I had found God through Jesus Christ. I confessed my sins to Jesus Christ - the most pre-eminent of which was my several abortions. I felt I had treated life too casually and repented. I had become a believer in God. One Sunday in September 1980 Kwabena and I had a terrific row. He told me I was nothing but a poor old woman incapable of doing anything constructive. I was devastated and determined to get a divorce. But I was pregnant and Kwabena was delighted about that. I began to get aches and pains and consulted my gynaecologist Alberto de Leon. He said there was nothing wrong. But I had a dream that my child was born dead. I had booked my air fare back to London for the beginning of December but before I went to the airport I was seized with incredible abdominal pain. At the airport I was incapacitated and felt I could not board the plane. An ambulance was called and took me to the hospital where the doctors pronounced me quite well. I went home with Kwabena but the pain was unendurable.

Kwabena took me back to the hospital where Alberto de Leon probed me for an ectopic pregnancy. He took me to the theatre to have a look at the foetus. I awoke from surgery unable to breathe and in deep distress. I was put on heparin for a clot on my lung and the pain in my abdomen was unendurable. I was in such agony that they had to clear the ward ,leaving just me in it. Alberto de Leon was exasperated. He said I was bringing all this on myself and he was sending a psychiatrist to see me. The psychiatrist duly came and spent five minutes with me. He said there was nothing mentally wrong with me and he had far more severely ill patients to see than to waste his time with me. To cut a long story short, I lost the baby and had a D & C. But I had haematoma and had to have regular treatment for this for some weeks to come. My miscarriage marked the final death knell to my marriage with Kwabena..

I stayed a little longer in Montreal to have a myomectomy - the removal of a large degenerating fibroid in my womb. Alberto de Leon felt I still had a good chance of getting pregnant again despite the fact that I was forty-six years old.

During this time I had a fateful meeting with an Australian dentist called Bill Webb. He became a powerful influence in my life. He showed me an alternative way of looking at things especially my marriage which was causing me a great deal of distress. He introduced me to the concept of vampirism whereby an individual would drain another of psychic energy by wounds and barbs.. Bill's knowledge was esoteric, seeking what lies behind the scenes. He had searched for many years and was still searching. He had practised as a dentist, but had given up this profession in favour of writing and painting. He was engaged to be married to a new found friend of mine Gretel Johnson, a Guyanese nurse. She became somewhat jealous of my relationship with Bill but it did not put a stop to our sessions of technique and learning. Bill introduced me to the works of Carlos Castaneda. I read the "Second Ring of Power " in February 1981. This was the most moving book of my life and I experienced ecstasy in reading it. It revolved around a yaqui way of knowledge which described warriorship and magic. I subsequently read all of Castaneda's books which became a guide to my way of being.

In March 1981 I left Montreal and returned to London. My twin sons Leon and Adrian and I resumed our stay at our family home "Prescott" in Palmers Green. I told them both of the rebirth I had experienced in Montreal and Leon took it up enthusiastically while Adrian had no interest in this aspect of my life. Adrian was very difficult and in trouble with petty crime. Leon had failed his A levels and took a year's sabbatical during which he developed an interest in computers and subsequently went on to take a computer course at Hatfield Polytechnic. Leon still today is in the computer business. Adrian had become an electrical apprentice but refused to study for his Guilds Certificate. Despite this he became a proficient electrician but caused much disruption at home, His girlfriend Sarah had also come to live with us and I treated her like a daughter. In the following year 1982 my daughter Chantal arrived from freetown with her three year old son Kemi and so we had a household. At this time Leon met Kerri who spent much of her time at "Prescott" but I never imagined that things would get serious between them. "Prescott" was a hive of activity. My friends, and the children's, coming in and out. But I was living on social security and finding things hard.

I already had a premonition that I would lose my home. I had property in Sierra Leone but this was not going smoothly. Donald Smythe-Macauley a long standing family friend was looking after my interests but his efforts were to no avail. I sold a substantial property in Leones (the local currency) instead of sterling due to Dom's inefficiency. This largely meant that we had to spend the money in Sierra Leone as the exchange rate was inimical to sterling.

In 1981 I joined the Rosicrucian Order based in California. They sent out monthly monographs which I read and studied avidly as did Leon. They were essentially metaphysical teachings showing how to open the psychic centres. I practised the exercises and in 1982 I had my first out of body experience. I awoke and felt as if I was having a heart attack. My astral or dreaming body was struggling to get out of the physical and managed to do this. My astral body reached the door of my room, opened it, and there was the ghostly body of a little child on the other side. I was so afraid I slammed straight back into my body on the bed. From then on astral projection became an habitual occurrence in my life. I also taught myself how to read the tarot and became very immersed in the archetypal images of this great mystery.

However I was depressed. I put this down to the fact that I had no money. I had tried to go back to teaching Economics and accepted a post at Barnet College. However when faced with the students and the blackboard my knowledge dried up and I found I could not remember my economics . The students liked me but I had to leave, that part of my life was over. I had taught Economics for twenty years very successfully both in Sierra Leone and in London. This was now over.

I read extensively, Ouspenski - all his works especially " In search of the Miraculous" inspired me. As did Elizabeth Haich "Initiation". But my greatest teacher was Carlos Castaneda. Second to him was Bill Webb who wrote me searching letters from Montreal and I responded tentatively at first, but then with more determination as my own understanding of metaphysics grew. However depression was a problem and by 1982 I was suicidal. I was persuaded to go to a Rosicrucian seminar in Sussex Greenwood Gate in October 1982. I arrived with great difficulty and saw this short Blackman. I thought Oh no, surely I haven't paid all this money and come all this way to hear a West Indian. So much for racial equality. Imagine to my amazement this man was dynamic - I fell in love with him reiterating later that God had spoken at Greenwood Gate. His theme was alchemy of spirit. He pointed out that what happened in the laboratories of the world also happened in the psyche. Human beings had tremendous potential but no way could they progress from one state to another without going through the dark night of the soul. Onslow Wilson mesmerised me; when I stood within his aura I could feel his vibrations and was electrified by them. I also met three women whom I found extremely stimulating: Leane Grimshaw, Deana and Muriel Henderson. We had a great time, and I came alive that week. But alas I had to go home.

When I reached home Adrian had decorated my room and all was harmonious. Leon brought me magic mushrooms - the first time I had taken mind expanding drugs. I played Oxygene and Gregorian chant on tape while I tripped. The trip was incredible. I saw God as everlasting truth infinitely revealed and I saw him as a dealer of cards. It was a kind of poker game in the skies. We were dealt five cards two of which we can change for better or worse. Then we must play with our hand as impeccably as possible. I also had a vision of the sphinx. The eyes where stupenendously beautiful and watching me. I also saw a slavering bear and felt a very bright light coming from my left. However it was too strong for me to look at. I also saw life size figures of Gog and Magog revolving in total symmetry.

I already had a premonition that I would lose my home. I had property in Sierra Leone but this was not going smoothly. Donald Smythe-Macauley a long standing family friend was looking after my interests but his efforts were to no avail. I sold a substantial property in leones

14

instead of sterling due to Dom's inefficiency. This largely meant that we had to spend the money in Sierra Leone as the exchange rate was inimical to sterling.

In November 1982 I had an anaphylactic shock, a combination of pain killers and alcohol. The painkillers were subsequently withdrawn from the market. I was in a lot of pain and decided to go to Newcastle to visit Muriel Henderson my Rosicrucian friend. She proved a great source of comfort and inspiration to me and by the sea I experienced a healing process. Muriel and I visited one another on a fairly regular basis for a few years and our friendship lasted until I became chronically mentally ill when it ceased. I had a few friends visiting at "Prescott" though I had already embarked on what was to become an increasingly solitary path. My creativity had been activated in Montreal 1980/81 and I did most of my writing in this period not all of it metaphysical. I did start a text book in "A" level economics which I never finished.

That which I dreaded came upon me and in July 1983 I had to sell "Prescott". I gave Adrian a deposit for a beautiful two bedroom flat in Bounds Green. Chantal obtained a reasonable council flat in Arnos Grove and Leon and I had a department of transport flat at Pymmes Close right on the north circular.

There was great sorrow all round at leaving our home. Kerry and Sarah were particularly inconsolable. But I could no longer afford a four bedroom three reception house which needed a lot of work. It had been magical while it lasted despite confrontations and conflicts. But now Leon Kerry and I took up residence at No 1 Pymmes Close. We all settled down quite amicably despite the tremendous noise from the north circular.

I visited the College of Psychic Studies in Kensington at

fairly regular intervals to glean some insight into my personal predicament of depression. I was told repeatedly that I had a good future. I had also consulted Mir Baslir a quite well known palmist in 1981 and I named his tape Life Line. He predicted a golden future for me including a third husband, a life in the artistic world and a prestigious position in a voluntary metaphysical organisation. He told me I'd have a lot of money in my own right and publish successful books. I often played his tape when I was feeling down. I subsequently destroyed it when I became mentally ill, but that is another story.

Leon and I had become especially close for we were both on the path together. Leon filled me in on scientific mode of esoteric knowledge, and I would feed him knowledge on the work I was doing which was largely ontological and epistemological. I was fired into writing. Much of it was in the theory of vampirism but there was much else on alchemy catalysts and peak experiences.

Pymmes Close was a hive of discussion and an experiment on omenology. I watched moths and birds and the skies and read into them for what was to be and what was occurring underneath the obvious. One day a deaths head moth materialised in the kitchen and we all knew a crisis was ahead. Moths materialised in the maisonette in the middle of winter and Carlos Castaneda had stated that knowledge was a moth. I had a friend Ann Cummer Price who had read "Tales of Power" and rang me to say she knew precisely what the moth meant. I wasn't to know but she was having a psychotic experience which I interpreted as a mind expansion. For suddenly she knew everything. Why things were arranged on a table in a particular way, why we thought as we did. And I marvelled at her experiences not realising she was ill. She recovered but went into depression which was hard to bear. She eventually recovered and denied all her experiences in an altered state.

Ten years later she again had a psychosis and saw space beings and colour therapy and reincarnation. But again she recovered and denied her experiences. Though this time she did not become depressed. She now lives a full and meaningful life with her husband.

I was very creative at Pymmes Close. I wrote an article "Black or white- the half caste's dilemma". This was originally written for a proposed magazine called Synergy which Bill Webb was initiating. He rejected the article as being too cold and intellectual. I subsequently showed the article to an Oxford don who said it was too emotional.

Anyhow I wrote a lot mostly along on ontology and epistemology. I also began a book called "The Race Odyssey" which described interracial dynamics in this epoch. I was trying to get an inquiry into half castes and their dilemma launched and applied to the G.L.C for funding. Paul Boateng dismissed my work but Peter Pitt liked it and only needed his racial inspector's approval to launch it. Unfortunately she classed my work as racist and nothing came of the project. It was a very disappointing time especially as I'd invested so much energy into the work. After my first psychosis I tried to get "The Race Odyssey" published but received six rejections and thereafter became too ill to peruse publication.

Leon and I became very close and shared much together. Unfortunately Leon had me on a pedestal which was to prove disastrous when I became both actually and chronically ill. However we enjoyed one another's ideas and inputs. Kerry at this time was very much in the background. She was depressed and feared that Leon did not love her as much as she did him. I encouraged her to develop, taking her to the College of Psychic Studies where I went quite often. I must admit that I no longer have faith in psychics - they all promised me a splendid future which never materialised. Kerry didn't find them useful either and in the long run neither did Leon.

I studied hard reading Carl Jung , Ouspensky , and above all Carlos Castaneda. I did meditation. I had taken the transcendental meditation course started by the Maharishi in 1981 and had a mantra but found this didn't work too well with me. I practised visualisation but this didn't seem to work either. I acquired the "Sixth and seventh book of Moses" and used the psalms for my various rituals but this didn't seem to work either. Where was I going wrong? I did magical practises in the rather extensive grounds of Pymmes Close. I did candle gazing, but above all I wrote and read. I also did extensive art work mainly montages which I called Lavatory Art; Madonnas next to whores, Bishops next to lavatories and I also did charcoal drawings. I was gradually becoming a recluse. I had one good friend Joya who was half Bengali and half Swedish and a medical practitioner. We spent many an animated evening together discussing life and metaphysics.

Chapter Two

In 1984 Bill wrote to me to tell me that he'd met a man called Ian Borts a trance medium who channelled entities called The Speakers Their philosophy was that each one of us was God and totally in charge of our destiny. I was appalled and wrote him a letter telling him how erroneous all this was. I said "I'm God, but what about all the other Gods around me who have the power?" Bill also sent me a transcript of a session he'd had with The Speakers. Shortly before this, Joya's mother Rosemary had passed me two Seth books which I cursorily read and promptly put in the dustbin. I felt they were too inherently evil. Anyway I was planning to go to New York to meet up with a friend called Carla Field. I spoke to Bill and suggested we meet in New York. In April 1984 I went to New York and stayed with Carla. Alas I couldn't bear it. Carla was living in a very primitive state and her morals left much to be desired. I telephoned Bill and asked if it would be convenient for me to come to Montreal. He said yes gladly, so off I went on to Amtrak and felt I'd arrived home when I got to Montreal. Bill and Gretel were in the middle of a divorce so things weren't entirely easy. Bill was full of The Speakers and gave me a tape to listen to. I did, but fell in to a deep sleep half way through. On waking I suspected the tapes were hypnotic.

I must admit to being utterly enthralled by The Speakers' knowledge which spanned almost every aspect of human experience. I fell in love with them despite the fact that I disagreed with their basic principles. These were that we alone create our world and everything in it. We create our friends, enemies and those in-between. We create our time and our seasons, we create our problems as stepping stones to our profit; we create our world and everything in it. But if each one is creating our own world, what about the

19

enormous conflicts that this would create amongst us. In any case my question was always which I is it? the conscious, the subconscious, or the supra conscious. Their dynamic was that we are all masters. They did a lot of work on mastership and its different grades : Force 1,Force 2 ,Force 3, and Force 4. Though they stated that a force 4 master would not overcome a force 1 master and all he had to do was run. Ian Borts himself ran his own workshop not under trance and talked about people's focuses. People had a predominantly physical, mental or emotional focus to their lives. But I later added the spiritual focus as in religious orders and New Agers.

Anyhow Bill and I were getting ready for a spiritual weekend which was to be held just outside Montreal at Contre Coeur. We had to make white gowns bearing a spiritual concept. Bill had Synergy woven on his gown which was the magazine he was to launch. I had "Apocalypse Now" with the sun underneath. Bill was in his element with young women gathering round him and flattering him. I was secretly furious for I was his Galatea and he was my Pygmalion. It was Bill who had awakened me to the truth and these young women were vacuous. But Bill had his brains in his balls and elevated these young women to force 4 masters.

At the spiritual weekend I was both attracted and repelled by Ian Borts. His power was undeniable and I could feel his vibrations at a very high frequency. He was avoiding me and a friend Rita said he was afraid of me for I could see right through him. He gave us readings of our auras and mine was double gold - his was double green and Bill's was double blue. Ian Borts proceeded to do an annihilation job on double gold and double blue. He stated that double gold denied themselves and were only interested in helping others and they were inimical to double green.

I took this as a warning off signal. He said that Double Blue were prone to addiction. Ian Borts was on a field day of power dominance.

When he relaxed into mediumship allowing "The Speakers" to come through things were much more relaxed. The Speakers held one session asking each one of us what we wanted. I said I wanted the gift of life, they replied by saying I should watch and wait observing everything and the miraculous could happen. Ian Borts asked us all what dreams we'd had the night before after placing a stone and a leaf under our pillows. I was pushed into giving my dream by Bill. Basically it was that a dog was tied on a bridge barking to be free. Large buses and lorries were hurtling over the bridge but the dog seemed unhurt. I felt sorry for the dog and went to release it, but as I did so the dog became more feline and sinister and I wondered what I would do with it at home. My recounting of the dream brought a lot of activity among the group, and an American psychologist took me aside to explain the dream to me. What I didn't voice was that I'd had another dream where Ian Borts was planning to leave his wife Rosemary and was searching in drawers and cupboards. I was standing by helping him.

The weekend was memorable and Bill and I returned to Montreal and Gretel. The latter said she had fully expected that Bill would announce his plans to marry me. I told her there was nothing of that nature between me and Bill.

I spent a lot of time trying to listen to The Speaker sessions and while I was copying one tape a strange thing happened. The tape went into reverse and a strange voice in a strange language superimposed itself on the tape, I was, to say the least, startled. and called Bill to come and listen. He suggested we take the tape to Pamela a psychic who was very close to Ian and his wife Rosemary. But when we took the tape to her it ran clearly with no other voice on it. I was puzzled. Anyhow I was preparing for my own personal session with The Speakers. I devised several questions. I asked first of all who am I?. They answered by saying that I was a powerful soul with incarnations associated with the Druids and Essenes. They said my great strength was also my greatest weakness - divine persistence. I quote "when the mind is geared and in motion there isn't a single force in the universe that can stop you, but often you will persist in things that are counter productive". I told them I was alone and incomplete and could a mortal mate with a God so that I could know even as I am known. They replied indeed yes, but completion is an inner process and cannot be achieved by a mirror image for often we see our wrinkles when gazing into the mirror. The whole session was very interesting but they were basically doing what they did with everyone inflating me. I asked them if they would come to London and they answered that they would be in the region of London in October 1984.

I returned to London in May in time to give Leon support for his forthcoming A level retake. I was excited, I'd bought their philosophies and hoped I could work with them in the future. However I'd lost my voice which had never happened to me before. Leon too fell into a deep sleep on listening to a speaker tape but he was interested in their work though not as extremely as I was. I kept on playing the tape " Clearing the mental picture" which had the voice in the strange language superimposed on it trying to work out the message. All to no avail it remained a mystery.

I was excited by the fact that soon The Speakers would be in London and I made some attempts to organize a welcome. However they, or rather Ian Borts, never turned up. They were liars. At around this time I asked my dreaming body to reach The Speakers to obtain more information in metaphysics. Immediately I was attacked in my bed, my face and chest paralysed. I couldn't breathe. I called on Jesus Christ and Mary to help me and I was eventually released. But in the meantime my astral body had projected me into the living room which turned upside down together with a religious stained glass window in one corner. Joya was there and said "surely The Speakers could not have done this to you, they like you".

From that time till my first psychosis in 1987 I was periodically attacked at night. My astral body usually projected seeking Leon's help. But on one occasion Leon was lying in a coffin and had the beak of a bird. I was so afraid I screamed. I then went to my mother but was told that she was sending the entity. My dreams were becoming infinitely more weird and became more real than my waking life.

Bill and I continued our high powered correspondence. But his letters were not as pungent as they had been before meeting Ian Borts and The Speakers. He was completely under their thrall and I was, to say the least, irritated by his submissiveness. I admit to playing the speaker tapes on a fairly frequent basis. They were filled with information and I was trying to glean some truth from them. I could not technically find fault with the teachings, but sometime in 1986 it struck me that they had no compassion. In addition they spoke a lot about the manipulators in our lives and advised that we get rid of them. Well this surely meant we get rid of everyone close to us. Marriages failed, children left their parents and as Bill came to acknowledge it was a veritable Jonestown.   .

In 1986 Bill acknowledged that he'd failed with launching the magazine "Synergy". He was also 30,000 dollars out of pocket with the venture. Not to mention the amount of money he'd spent on interviews with The Speakers. He wrote to tell me he was baling out and that he would subsequently tell me what was really going on behind the scenes. He said that this would make the Divine Comedy sound like a nursery rhyme. I, like an idiot, told him I was breaking off from all association with him and The Speakers. As far as I was concerned they had inflated all of us to take our energies into the unknown. They had described themselves as beings inhabiting an alternative reality where realities were created instantly. They had stated they had come to teach in order to move. Their friends had moved and they had searched the galaxies and not found them. But they needed to move.

Bill returned to Australia but was under constant siege from Ian Borts. He eventually returned to live with Ian Borts and co-operate in a book called "The Healer". In the authorship he had masqueraded as a doctor and apparently everyone in the Borts household called him Doc. But I am somewhat jumping the gun for in the meantime I was rapidly losing energy and became increasingly convinced that Ian Borts was trying to kill me and my children. This was possibly the beginning of paranoid schizophrenia. However I was paranoid and performed several ceremonies both for banishment and for protection. There was a protracted silence between Bill and myself but eventually we resumed correspondence.

Bill was very hesitant to discuss Borts and The Speakers though he did tell me that Borts was prosecuted in the Civilian Courts for malpractice. Bill said that Borts acted in an infantile manner and did his case no good. The courts found against Ian Borts and banned him from prescribing health cures through The Speakers. He ignored this injunction and continued to practise his transmediumship.

Chapter Three

I had become interested in the works of Maxwell Freedom Long an exponent of the K'huna method. He stressed strongly the relationship between the conscious, the subconscious and supra conscious. He stated that all the higher selves were in instant telepathic contact with one another. He stated the vital importance of being aligned with the subconscious and supra conscious. I gazed into my candle one night and asked for this connection. I went to bed and felt a click in my spine. I then experienced an orgasm electrically in reverse through my clitoris and was told by a voice that the subconscious wasn't where I thought it was i.e. it wasn't in the brain but at the base of the spine, the coccyx. From then on my writing in all directions flowed but I had not established contact with my higher self. In 1984 I also had a dream that I was going to the moon. I was settling all my practical affairs before flying. I was flying and nearly bumped into buildings. The dream had significance when in 1986 I had a dream that I had returned from somewhere and had lost my memory. I had a helper with me, but no one wanted to see me back.

I had three more trips on magic mushrooms between 1983 and 1987. In the first one I asked to see the devil. Imagine my surprise when I saw the beauty of artefacts, vases, floors, ornaments, all of immense extravagance. I eventually laughed and said Satan or Lucifer is the Prince of this earth. I had another trip when I asked for past lives. I saw myself as a priest in the middle ages, then as a black slave girl in the West Indies, then as a cowboy who's best friend was his horse, then as a Sudanese princess who was very rich and in love with her teacher. Her name was Farida and she cursed her wealth as stopping her from getting where she wanted. She was also having an affair with her brother Leon and I could not pass through the door where they were. In future in astral projection I was to call Leon my brother and not my son. I also had a vision of myself as a rather large extra terrestrial leaving those he loved behind and descending in a lift with six large eggs. The anguish I felt on leaving those I loved behind was indescribable. I was descending to earth the salt mines of the galaxies.

The next trip was a disaster. I saw the usual geometric signs but collapsed. I went to call for Chantal who was in the top maisonette and Leon was already there. I thought I was going to die. I saw Leon and Chantal as vampires and I was collapsing within. Leon kept telling me not to worry. My reply was that whenever a black man told me not to worry things were sure to collapse around me. Chantal eventually brought me out of my misery by telling me I couldn't lose self importance on my own. I needed witnesses. This occurred in 1986 the year my father died in Malta. I had felt his presence very close to me, but he had cheated me and my brother out of his inheritance. He had named his third wife Lina as usufructary of his estate exempt from giving an inventory. I tried to contest this from London but failed in my efforts.

The upshot was that I developed reversed airways and was admitted to hospital from where I was promptly discharged when I was found smoking a cigarette. My voice took several weeks to revert to normal. I had two dreams of my father. In the first one he was telling me that everything had gone wrong for him and he could no longer stay in St Paul's Bay (Malta). The second was he was redrafting his will in favour of myself. I told him it couldn't be done on the astral plane, it had to be manifest on the earth plane.

Pymmes Close had become a prison. I saw few people, though I saw Joya regularly. But I grew afraid of her due to a series of dreams where she was killing me. I had developed the habit of swimming three times a week, and I mastered diving which was a great achievement as I feared my head being underwater. I also went horse riding once a week. I was trying to keep fit, because physically I was out of shape. I was also emotionally drained with Leon providing the only emotional support. However he was becoming increasingly distant and more attached to Kerry. I grew jealous and late in 1985 I evicted Kerry from my home. Leon stated that if I forbade him to see Kerry he would comply. I answered that I would not forbid him. Kerry went to stay with mutual friends in Muswell Hill, Andre and Monica and Leon increasingly stayed over there at night. I could not bear what I saw as his betrayal of me and our cause and I asked him to leave Pymmes Close. Chantal was in the process of moving into the upstairs maisonette with her son Kemi so I would not be entirely alone.

In the meantime my friend Donald Smythe Macaulay came to visit from Freetown. I introduced him to the works of Carlos Castaneda for which he was grateful. He said he would always look after me, and was in the middle of an international deal that would have made him rich. He promised to buy me a new family house and give me a monthly income. Unfortunately his deal fell through and we remained poor. Don said he was worried at all the practises I performed at Pymmes Close without a teacher or guide. I felt like a walking laboratory. My aim was the Holy Grail, Nirvana, another world, cosmic consciousness . And yet I was becoming more and more depressed, and losing energy day by day.

At the end of 1986 I had an interesting experience. Castaneda under the tutorage of Don Juan had stated that some people had a double which was the self, but did not perform physical functions like eating or smoking. The double was capable of incredible performances. I was reading a Morris West book in bed. I can't remember the title but it revolved around a psychiatric patient of Carl Jung. It mentioned the God Janus who looked both ways and I had an emotive response to this. Suddenly my right side began to ripple and I felt a thump on my head. My double emerged and went straight to Montreal in seconds. I met some young people who offered me some food but I couldn't eat. Neither could I smoke when I tried to light a cigarette. I told them that I wasn't really there but somewhere else in bed. The problem was I couldn't remember where I'd left my body, whether it was in Montreal or London. I tried to get on a subway but couldn't board the train. Eventually I became very tired, and I looked on the full moon and asked her to get me back to my body. In seconds I slammed back into my body at Pymmes Close. The whole of my body was swollen with weals. I showed them to Leon and told him what had happened. I had a sense of well being following this incident.

I had been keeping dream diaries since 1984 and had developed my own symbology. Some dreams were very weird and interesting. I dreamt I was making a journey in pitch darkness with children , and did not know what I would find at the end of the journey if anything at all.

I dreamt that two magical sorcerers went through a kind of death in a motorcar, the chances of surviving were very slim. The woman survived, but her husband didn't. His face was handsome but wooden as she tried to kiss him back to life. I was watching and wanted to tell her that her attempts were useless. I dreamt that two black Dobermans deadly and indomitable vaulted down a staircase to kill. When they had performed their task they were gentle and docile on my lap. A white sheep dog who had lost his owner wanted to join us. I wondered how these dogs would get along but they seemed to settle down quite nicely in my car. I interpreted this dream as the Dobermans killing Ian Borts and the white sheep dog was Bill. Chantal and I often laughed when playing the speaker tapes and how sheep like Bill's questions were. Indeed all the study groups seemed mesmerised and never once challenged The Speakers. I had planned to challenge them on their proposed visit to London and in my writings was constantly aiming at topping their work. They had stated that though many cast aspersions to the conscious mind and that without the consciousness of ourselves we would not exist. I contradicted this dictum by stating that without the sub consciousness of ourselves we cannot live. And this proved correct when after my first psychosis I lost contact with my subconscious mind. I did not live, I merely existed on naked consciousness.

Through 1986 I wrote furiously and read avariciously. I went to the park about three or four times a week and went to feed the ducks, geese and swans. I described myself to my friend Bryony as Howard Hughes without the talons or the millions. I was becoming increasingly isolated, and broke off with my childhood friend Desiree Bellisario. She subsequently never forgave me for having sex with her ex husband Ray Bellisario the royal photographer. I noticed that I had started talking to myself out loud on the streets and worried about my mental well being.

In February 1987 I knew the end had come. I wrote my mother a letter thanking her for all she had done for me in spite of a very difficult relationship. I gave away the last of my jewellery to Bryony - a pair of Persian earrings in turquoise and ruby. I had already given away my rings to my band of young people. Adrian and Leon had mine and my first husband's wedding rings. Sarah had a wedding ring given to me by Bai Kamara a man in Sierra Leone whom I had hoped to marry. Kerry had my wedding ring from Kwabena and Chantal had my engagement ring from my first husband Ade. I called my grandson Kemi and gave him my miniature crystal ball for I knew I was going to die. I had also written a letter to Joya accusing her of trying to kill me through eye drops prescribed by her containing ephedrine to which I was allergic. I was entirely alone and in the grip of paranoid schizophrenia .

On the 13th February I was walking along the North Circular when my head split open. The noise of the traffic was horrendous. I entered my flat and someone knocked on the door, I opened it and a man asked for water for his car. I went to fetch it and then three men burst in and confronted me. They threatened to rape and kill me if I didn't give them money for drugs. I had no money and no strength to fight them even though I threatened them with a knife, I hid in the bathroom which didn't have a proper lock and I saw a vision of a beautiful kind woman watching over me. I called on her as my Mother to protect me and miraculously the men left the flat, though after emptying all my drawers and my bureau. I then went into a deep psychosis.

Adrian telephoned me to tell me that the car he had borrowed from me had seized up, the engine was finished. I laughed and he was surprised. My car's demise was just another aspect of my own death. Immediately I entered an altered state; The Speakers zoomed in communicating with me on beeps on the radiators. The noise was deafening. I bargained with them over quite what I don't know. But then I lay on my bed and my consciousness was bombarded by telepathic inputs. I was told of a speaker conspiracy to mutilate the world. The details were so horrific that I can no longer bring them to consciousness - but I asked for consensual agreement as to this conspiracy either from Bill Webb or Ian Borts. It was all too horrific. The entire area altered and became a wasteland. I was bled and my teeth were whitened and my eyes cleared. My fingers were implanted so I could communicate with the various energies manifesting themselves in my condition. My fingers clicked electrically with my every thought. Shortly before this episode Leon had become worried about me and took me to the Winners Club in Southgate where I had a sauna. My body did not perspire at all - it remained bone dry but my head perspired. In psychosis my body had been seized and was in the power of Saturn. I was told that I could have a new body more to my liking, and I fell for this. I started to specify the body I wanted. But in the meantime Hell manifested before my eyes. I saw it on the carpets beneath barren trees and hell fire. I was in hell. My brain was being bombarded by information which became too rarefied to bring back to consciousness. I watched the television and a black man came rushing out of the T.V to frighten me. I turned the T.V off.

The vision of the beautiful woman stayed with me. I told her she had no business being there in all that ugliness, but she remained for several days. I was possessed by a magician Hermes who was racing Ian Borts for another world. I saw the race on my blank T.V screen and the magician won. I was not alone, I had many other parts to myself. I was a cluster. The magician was a powerful aspect in my psychosis. I saw steam appearing at odd intervals in my flat especially the bathroom. The worst aspect of the psychosis was the physical torture I went through. As no one was touching me I can only presume that this was psychic torture felt through the physical body. My spine collapsed, I couldn't carry shopping , and had to leave my bag of shopping by the roadside. I was shrunk inside my body. The torture was unendurable. I telephoned for an ambulance one night telling them I was shrinking inside. . They didn't turn up. Chantal told me I should have told them I was having a heart attack.

Leon and Adrian discovered me a week after my psychosis began. Leon took me to St Thomas' Hospital. I was so panicked I fell to the floor and Leon was horrified.

When I eventually saw the psychiatrist he said there was nothing wrong with me and Leon wept. Leon tried to get me into the Arbors (a clinic set up by R D Laing) in Crouch End again to no avail. He eventually took me to my G.P who also seemed to think there was nothing wrong with me. But Leon banged the table and said something had to be done. So my G.P referred me to Chase Farm Hospital in Enfield. Leon took me there and I was admitted after crying in the waiting room that I had never been loved. What was also awful was that I saw everyone as a zombie or ghost not as human beings. I was admitted but escaped two days later. I didn't see the doctors as doctors, but as frauds and prisoners of the nurses. Dr Bench who was the consultant Dr Bowman's registrar and the only person I trusted. I went to see him at the Outpatients Clinic in Arnos Grove from time to time. I especially asked him to measure me as I was shrinking.

I carried on my psychosis at home. I was prescribed Stelluzine which I took. But all the while I was in a boat - a large ship which was planet earth. I was being hauled from the depths of the ship to the deck. In the meantime I was meeting my past especially in Sierra Leone, people I had known, and situations I had met. I was exposed. In the meantime the sick magician was possessing me and pleading for forgiveness for his sins. I prostrated myself on the ground outside my flat and asked for forgiveness. My collapsed spine was giving me a lot of stress and I couldn't explain it to anyone for no one saw any evidence of any torture.

Adrian took me to his place for a few days, and looked at me with great compassion but his girl friend Sarah couldn't cope with me and I had to return to my flat. While in the environs of St Thomas' Hospital my fontanel opened and my spirit escaped.

The pain was excruciating and I had to ask Leon for a scarf for me to cover my head. I had once dreamt that I was leaving this world through the top of my head. The physical torture was hard to bear but there were respites while I chatted with the Gods. I cannot remember the exact context of the conversations but they were very amusing and provided me with respite and a lot of laughter. The magician was always there.

I was told that I was part human, part animal and part robot and I should choose which of these I should be. I replied that all were equally valid, and I didn't care which I was. But food tasted of chemicals and I could eat very little. I lost weight rapidly. What shocked me that I was told that I was emulating the Christ myth and as I went to the shops I was being honoured as a Saviour. I felt this was blasphemous. Somehow I was saving the world, and I found that with other psychotics that we each felt we were special to the scheme of things. I was shown two worlds apart from hell. One was a metallic world which was very beautiful. The other was what I called the Ganges a world where the sun set on water and no-one was there apart from myself.

I stayed in those psychotic state for about three months and did not go back to the hospital despite Dr Bench telephoning Chantal to tell her I was seriously ill. At the end of the psychosis I collapsed. I needed a man desperately , not for sex but as a companion. I did not realise at the time I had lost my animus hence the desperate need for a man. I made a novena to the Virgin Mary to ask for a man and lo and behold I met one at the school where I had gone to do supply teaching.

My teaching was erratic and I was reeling from my recent

experiences but I could not bear to stay in my flat alone all day. I met John Wilkinson, a half Austrian teacher who took a fancy to me. We met on a few occasions and I had sex with him once. He offered to marry me and wanted to move in with me. But somehow I read warning signals and refused his offer. I still wanted my children to be close to me. However I was finding it hard to maintain any kind of life style and had drifted into clinical depression with internal tremors. By July 1987 I gave up the struggle and admitted myself into Chase Farm Hospital. I needed human company - any company would do. While I was still in the flat I met a Tony Cornell affiliated to the Edinburgh chair for psychic research. He said he found no evidence of negative influences either in my flat or in myself. However he would give me whatever I wanted. I interpreted this to mean sex, and though I was attracted to him I couldn't bring myself to ask him for sex. He visited me a few times but when I became severely depressed he backed off and broke all association with me. I had also joined Date Line and had met and dated a couple of men which proved fruitless. I was desperate for a man and searched around all my friends for one. The truth was that my animus had died and my spirit had left me.

I spent six weeks at Chase Farm in a very miserable state. I longed for affection and attention, and at the same time I longed to die. I begged Leon to bring me a gun so I could shoot myself. Prior to being admitted I had tried to go to an art class in Edmonton, but had to flee for I could not bear the company. I longed to be with people, yet with them I was alienated. I tried telling this to the staff in Suffolk ward, but they were indifferent. Indeed they were downright cruel with one nurse threatening to remove my bed if I kept on lying down on it. Leon had given me "Communion" by Whitley Schreiber which I read. On the fly leaf he had written with love and faith Leon. Leon couldn't believe I'd sunk under and wouldn't make it. By the end of six weeks I was abruptly discharged by Dr Bowman my consultant and I was faced with my flat alone. I was empty and wiped out and was afraid my children would desert me. However, I was admitted to Chase Farms' day hospital where I went by ambulance every day. I could not imagine how I had spent days all alone in my flat. I could not bear to be alone in my flat at this time.

By chance I met a young woman Debbie Herrick who adopted me. She was fascinated by me and looked after me. She did my washing and ironing and had me over at her flat. She was attending the day hospital for anxiety and panic attacks.

She became a fairly good friend and fell in love with Adrian .However Adrian did not fall in love with her and merely used her for sex. This was to prove fatal for our friendship. She was very attractive and a popular face in the hospital scene. We had some good times together. I enjoyed the day hospital where I met John McAleer one of the charge nurses. The attraction was instantaneous and I enjoyed our interchanges.

In the meantime I got a job at Network Education run by Francis Sealy. My work entailed running adult programmes. I had a good boss Mary Wheaton with whom I got on brilliantly. The job kept me going, and I met some very nice people there. What was really the highlight of the job was the lectures we were required to attend.

To my astonishment I met Morris Cohen who had run a therapy session at the Day Hospital at Chase Farm. He was lecturing in communications, but brought ontology and epistemology into the lecture. I was excited, his information was similar to what I'd been working on , and so I wasn't off course after all. Mo was pleased to see me and very excited by my comments in his lectures. At one stage he invited me to do the reading but I still lacked confidence. Debbie became infuriated that in that field I had stolen the limelight from her (I had obtained a job for her at Network Education) and turned on me viciously telling co-workers that I was mentally ill. I was furious and told her so. Chantal and Leon also warned her off her vengeance. The truth of the matter was that Debbie was suffering from Adrian's rejection and my intellectual brilliance which she could hardly match.

In the meantime Mo and I got closer and he said he couldn't come to terms with the fact that he'd met a mad teacher off the North Circular Road living in poverty and obscurity. Mo suggested we work together on training courses and I designed a course for him. He said it hadn't worked; well this was either because it was my course and not his own, or it was a lousy course. Mo and I spent many sessions together discussing metaphysics, ontology and epistemology and he was anxious that I got well enough to start work with him. I was deeply troubled when I discovered that his work wasn't his own but that of Werner Erhard of Est fame . Surely I'd have been better off talking to Erhard direct.

Chapter four

I was gradually getting better especially with the support of John McAllen at the Day Hospital whom I saw twice a week. I felt I was in love with John who told me that his wife found me a threat to their marriage. John refused to meet me outside the hospital and this was painful. In the end he was discharged for harassing a female patient. But our friendship had already ended at this time. John kept me going, as did also Chantal who spent every evening with me. I had a series of dreams where I was getting better, and I also felt a burning sensation paradoxically on the top of my head as if my spirit was returning. I also experienced a strange healing in my body which started from the inside. I had to roll on the floor to scratch my body.

In June 1988 I went to spend a weekend with friends Sue and Ted Killsy. I had known Sue for many years. In the middle of the night I awoke and felt great passion in my loins. I got up and writhed on the floor in an ecstasy of passion. I wanted to be penetrated, but not by a man. I was groaning in ecstasy. I was subsequently told by Dr.Dale Bechett a psychiatrist that this was a Kundalin experience. And it was the beginning of my next psychosis. The following morning I excused myself to Sue and Ted and headed home on the tube. I was well and truly spaced out. My head cracked and I screamed in agony. Chantal heard me and came to my flat to ask what was going on. My reply was I am part of an intergalactic engineering experiment.

I will now transcribe what I wrote in 1988 for my own benefit and in the hope that Chase Farm Hospital would as promised videotape it. The videotape never came to pass, but the following is an account of part of my psychosis which lasted for one year until July 1989.

After seven years of studying the science of being I acknowledge to being as mystified as Jung who states together with Carlos Castaneda that everything ultimately ends in a mystery.

Nothing metaphysically exists outside the mind (Nous); therefore all realities are contained there. The individual mind can contract , expand and shift perspective to include non-ordinary reality, for the natural world is only one mode of perceiving. Even in our solid practical world of reason there are incredible divergences of perception, politically, socially, economically and conceptually. The same disorder applies to the worlds of non-ordinary activity. No-one imagines anything. They may be confused to source or effect, but each conscious experience is real. Imagination relates to the activity of daydreaming visualisation or creating possible situations within the thinking function e.g. internal dialogues with oneself or another inserted in the script; imagining a satisfactory outcome or an ominous one in relation to hopes, wishes, plans, desires or fears. This facility is common to all normal human beings. I feel certain that each individual's "Walter Mitty" world cannot be described as madness but is indeed based on imagination or daydreaming. When a mentally ill person describes their experiences they are definitely not imagining them. They are too traumatised, depleted, confused, frightened to indulge in the leisurely visualisation that is used in a normal condition. Each patient's experience is real and misunderstood because it has not been shared, quantified or experienced by a majority consensus. Never dismiss the experience of the mentally ill as imaginary; it isn't. It closes therapy immediately as it is all too valid and actual and has a reason of its own. We are confused because we don't know how we've contacted these experiences or how they have contacted us or how to fit them into an ordered puzzle.

The mind cannot be seen or observed under any microscope - it is invisible. Therefore we are all dealing with an invisible, intangible, untouchiable and touching phenomenon, source or activity. The individual mind can only be observed as a three dimensional manifestation by our sensory experiences and our verbal communications. Additionally perceived by personal failure in satisfactory continuity with the social framework. Internally it is experienced as a breakdown in internal communications i.e .a confusion of inputs and very low or very high energy levels that are out of balance or spasmodic. In its extreme form the inner feeling is one of death, inertia and a desire for total loss of consciousness.

Verbal therapy can assist in re-establishing emotional validity and contact. (I am not here discussing emotional upheaval or the neuroses which are a feature in some degree to all living organisms - but only the type of breakdown which goes under the general title of psychosis). Contact and communication of all kinds is vital to psychosis or mental breakdown. Essentially each person needs to be re-catalysed. Each of us is a portable laboratory so that knowledge of chemistry is an ancillary to psychotherapy.

The separation of mind and body is impossible, for one's total body external and internal is the sole projection of the mind in the physical world. There is a sense in which the body is the mind when we are involved in the illness or its treatment. The nervous system is the main clue, the spine as the vessel of the autonomous, sympathetic and parasympathetic system is the matrix of the disorder and needs to be a focal point to the cure. For in our current state of lack of knowledge we must use the physical to combat the non physical. The brain is the central computer. Unfortunately only the brain studies the brain so we haven't got very far in knowing much about its workings and personally I have no new insight except to state that in mental disorder the brain has been attacked as though by a virus. As the 'physical' virus became known only in recent years, so it may be that in future research will be made in mental viruses invisible, but for me quite real. Again I have searched printed material and can find little information on the nervous system. Quantity unknown. Intuitively and corroboratively I feel that its sympathetic vibrations keep us in harmony, life and contact with the universe. Any damage here causes us loss of contact with life sources.

In the same way as foreign organisms internal and external attack the body and cause disease, so do similar intelligent organisms attack one's mind. Mental illness is an attack on the mind from an invisible vital source emanating from layers of mind realities to which we don't have access. For we all live in our usual consciousness. A vital clue that such an attack may be taking place is the nature of dreams i.e. nightmares. Isolation either mental or social is a key to being open to attack by the weakening of one's protective system. Work is being done on dreaming in laboratories especially in Russia and America which is coming up with some interesting findings. Embryonic work is being done in Britain too, but is generally frowned upon by establishment. I feel and hope that the next twenty years will see a revolutionary breakthrough to the entire mental health issue effectively making a break from Adler/Freudian tradition and greatly expanding the being. What on earth happened to Laing? We need tangible scientific tools to tackle mental breakdown, and these may have to include the existence of worlds or layers of life often called astral in the occult or esoteric world. We were reluctant to accept Chinese acupuncture in the fifties and today academia is reluctant to include the occult but it may have to do precisely that at some stage.

Occult in its pure meaning is hidden.

Back to the body which is the only tool that has been available to me during my illness. I suffered terrible panic attacks and did not know how they were triggered or how to stop them.I found them one of the most difficult symptoms of my illness. I was eventually helped by Carlos Castaneda's "The power of silence" where he spoke of the body having several points of assemblage. He states that these positions for altering one's state are definitely not in the head as most of us imagine, but in the body. Carlos

Castaneda has been my finest teacher and I would recommend that those involved with treating the mentally ill examine his works; if they only take from them the value and importance of one's body in altering states of consciousness or well being.

Anyhow I asked my body to shift its assemblage point from panic to peace. I asked my midriff section to close itself to stop energy loss and mounting fear. It worked, after some weeks of this repeated request I ceased to have panic attacks and though I have felt a lot of fear since, my mid section has nevertheless remained stable and closed.

I'm not a physiologist, so cannot digress in precise point triggers, but I do know that much mental disorder can be counteracted through attention both mental and physical in the miracle of one's body. For example therapy is fantastic, but so is sunlight, water, steam, fire and rolling on the earth, all elemental energy sources. I also know that quick thumps or jolts in the back and neck can re-align the spinal communication system. It's a form of controlled counter shock. I found that manual jolts also revitalized me when I felt dead ; the hands seemed to be high energy transmitters almost like the biblical laying on of hands.

The key to regulating the mental attitude and strengthening one's own energy fields is attention and this doesn't have to be verbal or visual contact all the time, but some focus that emanates higher energy frequencies into the phyche e.g. music comfort and reassurance. Spite of any kind is always counter productive - it drains energy the patient can't afford. Intelligent caring anger however can be highly effective.

The occult has a bad reputation but it exists; it encompasses mind and the invisible and is a concurrent to any psychology of the mind. Practitioners often refer to the occult simply as the subconscious. The latter has several layers and the deepest are connected to occult forces or powers which surround our world. This is true for all of us. It's just that up to now the norm has generally been to be unaware of these deep layers which can encompass infinity itself. The movies and literature of our time are evidence that people are increasing their contact with so called psychic centers and perceiving non-ordinary realities connected with both the subconscious and supraconscious mind channelled through the nervous system, registering in the brain and processed into the thinking and sensing functions. To deny this is to be an ostrich, and yet these abilities or internal voyages are still too much a minority experience to merit consensual acceptance in Europe.

My own mental illness emerged primarily and foremostly from my involvement with the occult, which was part of my field of studies on the science of being. I experienced the breakdown as an invasion of tremendous force into my mind, my body and my brain. I was frankly unprepared for the onslaught which felt like ritual murder. However I feel sure that this would not have occurred had I been living with other people - my isolation laid me open to attack and had also weakened me emotionally through lack of normal sensory stimulation - hence my psyche was not confident or ebullient. Confidence and vitality are excellent safeguards to dispel mental attack whether by a virus, a subconscious internal split (which becomes an entity in itself attacking the immune system - viz all auto-immune illness such as angio neurotic oedema etc is self versus self). Or another person being or entity who practises mind rape and body invasion. The symptoms of internal manipulation of organs are caused by control of the brain and nervous system by the attacking entity. According to which button is pressed, so to speak, all internal and external sensory perception is altered, reversed or travestied. Because only I can feel or see this or that, and no-one else can, it is all labelled hallucination, i.e unreal. Absolutely <u>not</u>, delusory it may well be, i.e an impermanent distortion of truth and balance, but hallucinating as in non-existent or imaginary it is <u>not.</u> Moreover the hallucination can also be perceptions of states of being not ordinarily available to us and therefore just as valid as our material taken for granted world. What remains a fact is that such an attack destroys the balance and energy of mind and body and psyche, and the danger is that the trauma or damage can be permanent unless there is found an appropriate antidote to restore oneself.

Chapter five

In my opinion current medication is merely a placebo and of negligible value. We must search for medication with plants - so called 'primitive' medicines. Beside the nettle grows the dock weed i.e. the antidote to the sting. I am not indulging in wishy washy alternative medicine mostly copied without any true medical understanding, from foreign cultures or hearsay. What I am advocating is a responsible review of the entire world of drugs many of which no longer work. We need to find truly potent remedies to re-establish body chemistry during mental illness. The structures of psychiatric wards are an inhibiting factor in encouraging nurturing through frequent hot drinks or cold drinks etc. Fluids ought to be available on tap so to speak. Dehydration can occur quite quickly with mental illness. I found that my body soundly monitored my intake needs, e.g .lots of fresh lemon, or lots of meat or no food at all. But in fairness, the human contact on the ward and its day ancillaries also saved my sanity.

The conspiracy of silence. Most of us never tell the psychiatrist or staff or anyone else the 'truth'. We feel like pariahs or untouchables, rape victims or the dregs of the earth. To be told we are mistaken or imagining or self pitying or not fighting hard enough or sick in the head, or any of the multiple put downs that our peers and carers place on us, firmly seals our lips. We then become liars, secretive patients talking to other liars - uncomprehending staff. There is a time to keep silent and a time to speak. When I began to speak of my trials and tribulations I met one person who had very identical experiences to my own though of less intensity. This person was intelligent and articulate but had never been believed and like myself went into hospital because she was scared of being in her flat alone. We don't speak up because we are trying to save a little of our pride and self esteem. I was asked by John McAleer to speak up and if my experiences would add to all of us concerned, it may after all not have been in vain.

I have labelled my illness metapsychosis as a convenient subdivision to existing labels. I feel that in the current and future trends this could be applied to other 'prevailing' cases, i.e. those who are questing meta knowledge and are fast increasing in number in all walks of life. It is increasingly being referred to by alternative thinkers and instructions in the fields of metaphysics and anthropology, philosophy and psychology. The works of Carl Jung and Ouspenski. also remain a major inspiration in my studies. Richard Bach, Maxwell Freedom Long, and Elizabeth Haich were also valuable. And through the seminars of Mo Cohen I realised that much of my work on ontology has much in common with Werner Erhard of EST fame.

I have already mentioned my return to Montreal in 1984 and my meeting with Ian Borts and The Speakers. On my return to London I played their tapes on a constant basis trying to discover their secret whereby they created their realities instantly. Their knowledge certainly transcended any that is normally available by man. They were able to be anywhere on our planet instantly, read any material in anyone's possession, see through the human body, know precisely about everyone in a kind of X-ray ability.

People flooded to Ian Borts for advice and medical cures. The output of personal and collective sessions was enormous and had a vast spectrum of knowledge, medically, metaphysically and psychologically. Ian Borts was making 'loads of money' and my Australian friend Bill was truly hooked by the affluence and promises that never actually materialised. Somewhere deep down inside despite my fascination with the knowledge, I felt Borts was manipulating and deceiving everyone. I also felt he hypnotised the subconscious mind.

I decided that both Ian Borts and his space beings were manipulations par excellence and by 1985 I broke all connections with them and my friend and tutor Bill.

The Speakers were liars and I'm sure were responsible for the paralyzing attacks I experienced at night. I continued my own studies of the paranormal. My dreams became increasingly lucid and were often bizarre. They became a major source of problem, psychologically and in establishing a coherent pattern of knowledge of the subconscious or the inner self. At many levels my dreaming was highly schizophrenic and had little or no relationship to my everyday reality. I had to throw out Freudian interpretation of dreams and indeed all other conventional interpretation of dreams. Eventually I came to the conclusion that the bulk of my dreams were programmed i.e. dreamt through me and not by me, as indeed I have intuited that the bulk of what has occurred to me has been programmed as though by a computer or demonic possession. In a sense all of this confirmed the force of destiny as distinct from that of free will and choice. I concluded that human beings could not be blamed or held responsible for their lives, which were determined by a force or power or will outside themselves.

Nevertheless my intent began to draw out dreams which were not programmed and I continued to have out of body experiences and travel great distance and partially know what others were doing or thinking, a form of sleeping telepathy which I called 'seeing'. Scientists now call it Remote Viewing and Russia has used this ability to know what occurs in America without the intervention of normal communications. My lucid dreaming showed me several facets of non-ordinary realities, and more relevantly what Ian Borts and his group were really up to. Briefly and as an overview he was bent on being a kind of God on earth as a healer, teacher and transmitter of extra-terrestrial power. But these extra-terrestrial entities were also planning to invade flesh and blood and mind and make us into zombies. We obviously had something they didn't have, and they were determined to get it. I saw that in reality they were mad mutilators, killing, maiming, raping and stealing under the guise of healing and helping. My logic and reason found all this hard to accept, yet my direct body knowledge and dreaming telepathy insisted that this was true. I was in a dilemma, who would I tell, who would believe me?

The plot thickened through mind expansion and seeing. I began to realise that I was genetically linked to their galaxy and was indeed similar to them in some way. I knew they had hoped to use me to spread their work and doctrine in Britain.   I had, and still have no-one to turn to for enlightenment in this and I thought of having sodium pentathol regression. This plan was however vetoed by Dr Bowman. The planet The Speakers inhabited was grey and highly mechanical, full of ghastly machinery. My daughter Chantal saw this on her one and only mind expanding experience. She also observed that spores were left here which were not supposed to be here and gave me additional clues to my now current nightmare on the nature of my own being. For I also saw that my brain was like a computer and unlike the 'norm' of the human brain. In hindsight I was in a delusory state for I also saw myself as an android and a splendid space being.

As I have already mentioned in June 1998 I entered another altered state despite great strides having been made in returning to health. I feel certain that my state was caused by highly intelligent devices that control the brain and nervous system and alter all physical realities or phenomena as we are ordinarily accustomed to them. Zigzag lightening strobes in my inner vision together with internal buzzing lead me to believe that the force is electrical in nature. I felt as if I was being cracked wide open. The suffering this time was not just human but also both animal and God like. It felt at one stage like the agony of a God.

All my nervous tension was loosened and I experienced feelings of hollowness. There was also extreme torture to the internal organs with sensation again of spinal and muscular collapse. Additionally there was writhing and twitching of face and body. My teeth became clean, and body odour underwent change. My hands again became impulsed but on this occasion there was no unseen force, it occurred spontaneously. My balance or specific gravity became impossible; small weights felt like lead and I seemed to change in size in different environments, at the time feeling like Alice in Wonderland. My feet felt as if made of metal and the strength in my hands was immense. I could easily bend metal and did so.(Through all this experience my three cats were composed, alert, aware, loyal, co-operative and very obviously also part of the 'experiment'). In fact I looked to their extra-sensory perception for guidance when I had none of my own. I had utter admiration for their intelligence and courage and what Castaneda called silent knowledge.

Chapter six

Ian Borts and The Speakers zoomed in again for a metaphysical competition. Again I gave out my knowledge under duress- much of what I gave out telepathically I was unaware of ever having known. It was knowledge on cosmology and I remember thinking that there was lots more to learn than I already knew. Unfortunately I was unable to remember my insights. Carlos Castaneda calls these states heightened awareness which are easily forgotten when we return to ordinary reality, similar to dreams that fade on waking. Much did hinge on the concept of the Eternal Now and the connection of the past, future, and present as a circular continuum. The gist again was that Borts was in some sort of control of me and had presumably via these space entities, been monitoring me for some time in order to either annihilate me or make an android copy of me elsewhere more to his physical liking. His attitude seemed ambivalent like love/hate. Briefly I told him to drop dead and that it was going to be my life or his, and it wasn't going to be mine. I'm strongly paraphrasing the battle and events, for a full account would fill a good sized book (indeed all my psychotic material has been paraphrased). The Speakers briefly congratulated me, for what I still don't really know. The main thrust seemed to be movement to another planet with a renewed solar system. This confirmed the information I had received in psychosis in 1987 that they and I via the magician were racing for another world before this one died in the Piscean Age . Fantastic, yes that's what I once thought but I retained an open mind on the subject particularly in view of my erstwhile esoteric studies which I had considered to be my own personal and inviolable designs. The latter seemed to have become against my will public property, and in my view were being used for the purposes of other forces or powers in the universe. I know of no other individual in the esoteric field who shared my own personal designs, explainable only in abstract terms. I am aghast that these entities, whoever or wherever, could prise them from me, steal them for their own benefit. I called it piracy and contravention of copyright in high technological places. For indeed it seems that our planet is only one of many worlds or universes in our galaxy. Moreover The Speakers' own universe had its own problems so two universes and solar systems were presumably involved.

Again sensory perception altered dramatically from day to day. At one stage everything became deathly quiet, not a sound from anywhere; this alternated with deafening noise from traffic and machinery. I can't explain the latter as I did not see the machinery that generated so much noise.

I was ritualized, taken back in consciousness to Methuselah so to speak, and relived myths and archetypes through the ages both telepathically and physically. On several occasions I felt sliced in half as though my back were missing My right thigh was paralyzed, my womb area manipulated and sexual abuse occurred. Much of what I experienced was humiliating especially as I was informed it was being filmed for realities in the cosmos, precisely where I don't know. I admit to seeing laser lights and chiaro scuro images on the walls of my flat. I laughingly informed them I was now a B movie queen and that God had better take care if this is what was going on in his cosmos, or the shit would, so to speak hit the fan. I asserted that my 'invisible' work was worth millions and fully expected to be paid. However I was then informed that this wealth was being diverted to copies of myself made in other realities. I called the whole lot of them criminal weirdoes and perverts. The threat to kill me completely was always present, as was the threat to impoverish ruin and annihilate me. Briefly it was three months of ritual drama whose detailed saga would be of interest only to students and teachers of the occult and paranormal. Dream realities were again bizarre most of them showing how many methods these beings had of killing me and isolating me, or more frighteningly turning me into an android who wasn't truly me and would be unable to walk or function normally. Inner visions and realizations were many; my eyes became hollow like windows with black worms emanating from them. The vision of colours changed, becoming intense as in pictorial art and my navel became hollow like a clay hole. By and large I judged the bulk of these sensations perceptions and realities both delusory (not illusory) and miasmic. I called them lies, infernal lies and demonic lies. The chanting of the Catholic Mass at intermittent intervals was supposed to be celebrating my death, and death seemed central to both my first psychosis and this second one i.e. my own death.

I was aware of many solid presences around me, pressing on me, pushing me or communicating with me. Some were people who are alive and I know, others like my father and grandfather who are dead. But all had some role or function to perform in this ritual drama. Particularly my dead family who seemed to be using me in some way as if they had sold me to the devil. My father particularly was as real to me as if alive, and seemed to be helping me to kill Borts. However, I had my doubts when I had a vision of my father Tony entrapping my brain on a T.V screen for his own ends. Later I saw he had entrapped me in a room which was changed by magic for ritual purposes to my disadvantage. My own private knowledge of my father and his lineage prompts me to believe some of this and now far from being proud of my unique ancestry, I had resolved to divorce myself from it completely and delete a name I was once proud of. There are indeed stranger things in heaven and earth than are dreamt of in our philosophy.

The battle with Borts was actually fascinating and as an equal being of flesh and blood I did not fear him at all. Throughout most of the stages I and my flat were lifted away from the entire environment as if by magic. I felt as if I was in the nagual a term used by Casteneda to describe another state physically by means of going through a crack in the world like the Bermuda Triangle. The essential feature of my being became sorcery or enchantment. My body became totally flexible, double jointed and tireless. My task was to enchant him and mesmerise him. This I did over days with hours of dancing, gymnastics and acrobatics which were impossible in my ordinary state, and till now leave me amazed as to how I performed such impossible physical .acts. For days I neither ate nor smoked. My only clue was that twice in dreaming I was able to act this way with a double body which I have called my dreaming body, and which feels as physical and solid as the one I am in now. However this double, as Carlos Castaneda calls it doesn't eat or drink or use the lavatory. In this instance my double became myself intrinsically combined. Adrian my son saw me performing and immediately left in horror. One other woman saw me performing and was fascinated. My feet could turn to face the opposite direction, probably I was a candidate for the Olympics. This is about the only aspect of my experience that I would like to reproduce, for the sense of well being in this super physicality was fantastic.

Mentally I also had to be right on the ball and play Ian Borts at a kind of glass bede game at all levels, knowledge, emotion and personal. Insults hurled around in plenty and the gist was that I told him I was going to chop him up in little pieces, break his fingers and see him in hell. Sexual dynamics abounded and I had great difficulty in fending off his efforts to seduce me. He told me he was in love with my mind. I can vouch that in that state mental and psychic seduction is more powerful than our ordinary face to face attraction. The mind which is invisible becomes as real and tangible a force as the physical presence.

I had to outsmart Ian on every aspect of creation, which

included communicating with the four lords of creation who hold the balance of the four corners of the world and the four directions. I had to whirl like a dervish for these so called lords to placate and reason with them to declare the fight in my favour. The force of Satan and his role on our planet was a frequent source of discussion. Ian told me I was the daughter of Satan with occult or divine privileges and concomitant disadvantages. In my normal state all this sounds quite bizarre, but at that time it seemed to have a grain of sense. Though I admit that I rejected ninety percent of what was said, telepathied or informed as totally false and delusory while it was occurring. I feel that on this occasion my continued denial and rejection of this rubbish actually got me through and out of that particular stage of metapsychosis. I pronounced it all evil, confusion and unintelligent miasmic nonsense. Nevertheless I had no choice but to participate. My mind was under seizure and control and it was clear that my challenge was to escape this control.

The God theme figured prominently throughout and I jokingly called Ian God on earth and finally teased him ironically to death, even writing him a pungent and sarcastic poem. Whereupon he dropped dead with an internal haemorrhage. This news was confirmed by Bill Webb in Canada. However this wasn't the end and I still had the entities to deal with, though I strongly suspect that they were linked with the force that was called Satan devising several ways to still kill me off. I caught a brief vision of myself and I looked awful. I also found that spontaneous orgasm fended off death and danger.

The intrinsic connection between my own family and Bort's also re-emerged i.e. that we were Karmically famililialy, or genetically linked with what I've called for years galaxy one thousand, the space entities' universe. When my

54

Australian friend confirmed Ian's death by phone I shed a few tears and prayed for Ian's soul; such is life and death and the game I've called roller ball, kill and be killed for dying takes many forms.

Externally the earth moved and turned; there was a change in my carpets. A burn mark had shifted its place which neither I nor my children could find any logical explanation for. Anyway the flat revolved and my cats and I were ecstatic. The air was fresh, the sun shone, and everything including the traffic moved more slowly. My flat became instantly clean and fresh smelling with everything shiny and sparkling. The oven grill cleaned itself; this was fairyland indeed. My clock behaved strangely, racing; six hours seemed only like six minutes. I thought so here's the experiment with time which I'd been informed about; back from the future. For so much seemed to turn on this illusion of time and eternal recurrence. I was asked to save several people from hell and list the cosmic work I had performed. These were abstracted from my flat as was indeed so much else. I was informed that we had made the transition to a new sun and a new world from one millennium to another. My cats were obviously undergoing physical changes and I intuited they were being alchemised. They were happy, calm and aware. However this state of euphoria didn't last for it was followed by a sudden change.

The flat again became hell, cold as a tomb, fetid and with sounds of dripping water. The walls were hollow and my body deteriorated especially my hair which became lifeless. My nails grew overnight and were hard and tough and collected inexplicable dirt. In fact my physical changes throughout this time were enormous, as were my emotional and mental states. All three were agonizingly unstable and would vary drastically daily. Galaxy one thousand maintains to be able to alter and manipulate all physical phenomena instantly. If one adds to that control of the

55

brain and nervous system, then the mind and emotion can be played with similarly to playing a piano.

Again I had to fight for my life with beings who called themselves 'higher selves', i.e. guards or guardians on our astral plane who would prefer to be physically in a body. Occultists and metaphysicians are usually aware that many ethereal or quasi-solid forms of life long to be in the flesh and will do anything to get a body if they can. I have never discovered what it is about flesh and blood that is so special or unique in the cosmos; but it is a mystery; hence the sacrament of the body and blood of Christ. For indeed I do believe that there are manifold forms of life in the so called invisible worlds as there are in our physical world. Anyone interested can refer to the mathematician P Ouspensky's "Tertium Organum" or "New Model of the Universe". These propositions and abstracts seem strange or imaginary to the majority of mortals because only a minority till today quest meta-knowledge; as only a few pursue the fields of astronomy or atomic energy.

Eventually I fought my way out of hell and rejected all entities who were trying to possess my body. Many of these entities were named and I told them all to die and get their worlds and realities destroyed.   I announced "Apocalypse Now" at large to every world or being presented to me.   A vision of one of these worlds was amazing, colourful as rich renaissance, not beautiful, but all everyone seemed to be doing in it was enjoying themselves and having sex and eternal youth.   After a few minutes I asked for the vision to be removed, it was exhausting.

Then for a period my flat was littered with rubbish, matches, cigarette stubs and everything was instantly teleported. Money vanished instantly from my purse, as did plates and clothes. The plants began to move, their leaves tapping me in the head. I was so frightened I threw all the plants away. Simultaneously cloth and clothes and curtains also writhed and moved and refused to keep still on my body.

My cats clawed frantically at them. My state of disgust and amazement was indescribable. I had to throw out most of my clothes in bin liners and almost immediately grubs and bugs leapt out of the bags. My cigarettes and matches were constantly removed, my tarot cards moved and played with and countless other phenomena which normally could only be effected by a human being. However these phenomena were happening without human energy. Yet my cats were constantly chasing and smelling these presences, on the carpet, in cupboards, behind gas fires and at the windows. I could see nothing but felt forces powerful all around me causing me pain and distress. A bag of stone runes was thrown outside and the pieces scattered under a tree, though the rune of destruction was left under my bed. Throughout my body was in a state of collapse like a puppet or android gone wrong.

Explosions began to occur through the floorboards, and horrible bloodless unearthly insects emerged from the floors. I killed most of them but kept a sample of one, crustacean, odd and bloodless. The main thrust of this seemed raw naked power and the ability to animate so called lifeless matter or generate it from what had already died. The saga felt like 'Nightmare in Elm Street' parts one, two, three, four, five and never ending. At one stage I felt ghosts banging on me in bed and was hoisted round the flat in pitch darkness floating like a banshee.

This primitive horror was in direct contrast to the high technology involved in teleports and subsequent phenomena. My cat Isis was teleported then thumped back into the flat, while my own consciousness jumped intermittently from one reality to another as if the area I lived in had a similar parallel and another self identical to me. I found clothes in my washing machine that I had not placed there and did not belong to me. As my consciousness jumped from one self to another I tentatively concluded that maybe we had a twin planet. I was constantly under pressure to prove my identity and unity with myself on the basis of consistent aims and desires and memory of my past. Till now I remain in wonder at such an experience and have no logical explanation. However Ouspensky again proposes that a twin self in a twin planet is metaphysically feasible. There seemed to be slight differences or discrepancies between the two flats and areas between which I fluctuated. On the other hand, it is possible that I was in a time warp and that my experience is confined only to myself and does not involve any other part of my world or that of others. For indeed the significance of time recurred right through and the information that I was caught up in a time warp. But I admit to not understanding this despite the fact that at one stage I went backwards in time from the twenty second September back to the sixth. I remained on the sixth of September for three days and then went forward normally to the twenty-second September. These shifts occurred during brief periods of loss of ordinary consciousness, a kind of dream coma. However I did not have a black out and was not at all times too aware of what occurred.

It seemed as if two forces were constantly competing on their abilities to provide benefits for planet earth and on animating so called dead matter such as cloth or lower forms of life such as plants and insects. Moreover I felt like a battlefield for an intergalactic engineering experiment and my body did not feel right, as if there were a hybrid problem.

I would have been prepared to dismiss this as purely personal had it not been for the fact that my radio cassette,

T.V and video recorder were totally altered. None of these machines had ever had particularly good reception. To my amazement the sound on my radio amplified and became crystal clear; the green and red lights switched on in harmonious vibration to the sound; they hadn't previously worked. A multitude of stations became available which before and later were not available. Broadcasts were also in strange languages. But what was funny was the short interposed announcements on what Canada was doing. "Keep your brains well wrapped up when going to Canada". It was unfortunate I couldn't record and film all that was happening. I asked John McAleer for a video camera but he didn't have one. I also asked him to come and verify these broadcasts at my flat, but I guess for professional reasons he could not come. No one else would stay in my flat long enough to be able to give consensual confirmation of transmission both on radio and television.(Incidentally for much of the time my telephone was out of order).

Special broadcasts were given throughout on channel two and four interspersed with normally listed programmes. There were too many to detail but the gist was political movements of the future, the interpretation of past events in history, the racial issues, technology and send ups of what the Borts group were doing, i.e. daydreaming of changing the world to no effect. The broadcasts which I cannot explain kept me going with their sanity. Moreover skits and scripts were shown on the nefarious plot of galaxy one thousand to make androids out of human beings leaving us as zombies.

One 'final' showing made me ill and shocked. It was shown in October 1988 at six am on BBC2. My space being floating in to space towards a warped sun that looked like a raped embryo; two masked surgeons operating on an unseen patient and simultaneous clippings of Humphrey Bogart, saying " play it again Sam" strange medical remedies and foreign meteors. It was like a photo montage with no sense or sequence. All this caused me to have horrific visions of people and phenomena I can't describe for they are alien to my consciousness. I was also able to see through my closed lids.

I was immediately exorcised by the Roman Catholic Diocesan exorcist; I was crying and afraid as my whole body shook with ghastly visions in deep red and black passing through my mind and going as if into distance or eternity. The Westminster Diocesan exorcist together with other members of the Catholic Church were proficient throughout and I felt that without their intervention my condition would have deteriorated. I also received healing from the monastery Vita et Pax at Oakwood.

My flat was also exorcised but was then twice robbed of most of my durable goods, television set, video, washing machine, furniture and personal jewellery. The bathroom was desecrated by the thieves. My cats were traumatized and I dared no longer sleep there. I received asylum at Chase Farm Hospital. A further personal exorcism was performed on the fourteenth of December 1988.

At one stage during my backward time warp my vision altered so dramatically that the skies became vast and far like oceans. I felt sea sick and almost as if an ocean from the, sky was going to collapse onto earth. Strangely I also smelt sea water and the theme that our planet was like a ship immersed in an ocean recurred intermittently throughout my experiences. I then thought of the biblical flood.

World weather underwent changes in this period, the Jamaican, Mexican and Texan hurricanes being the most startling. My body and mind were not functioning normally nor was my vision with lids closed or open. I still felt under control and was struggling to dispel the invading forces. I labelled my experience the most horrendous crime in the cosmos, the unpermitted invasion of mind and body and the exploitation of my brain by these entities whether from our galaxy or another. Additionally my outside environment changed fairly dramatically to my own perception during my time warp. Everything became very clean and renewed looking, but strange objects popped up, like old carpets embedded in the grass, nineteen thirties type machinery in adjacent wastelands and the blossoming of fantastic blackberries, plants and flowers. New shop fronts appeared while old ones disappeared. But throughout there were no other people in sight, nor any cars, everything was deathly silent. I couldn't see any of my children during the time warp; they disappeared.

One morning police came to arrest me while I was lying down exhausted and frustrated in the back garden of a cottage. I had thought that the surrounding environment was enchanted and that people and children were imprisoned behind magic glass. I had tried to break the windowglass of the cottage to release the prisoners. The police told me they had an ambulance waiting to take me to hospital for they knew I was mentally ill. Earlier I had seen a policeman on the corner of my road speaking into a walkie talkie. I was petrified and quickly prayed to God that I wouldn't be seized and taken into an ambulance. Believe it or not, the policeman instantly vanished and I saw no sign of an ambulance. This was the most significant instance of people or objects vanishing in my environment; there was another occasion when my daughter vanished before my eyes. Is it possible that I exchanged universes in consciousness from this reality to its twin.

The underlying theme during my time warp was that I and others had parallel selves in an identical planet and it was I who was shunting backwards and forwards between the two. It was very disorientating to say the least. And then I wonder whether my twin self was sitting in an identical hospital writing all this down as I was doing then. Carlos Castaneda makes many references to double and parallel beings, and I suggest that if anyone is interested in my experience they read through his works which are among the best sellers in the world and quoted by the scientist Kapra.

I must also mention that my ordinary cassettes did not play what was on them, but music that was alien and superimposed; it was haunting and beautiful and I called it space music. Additionally a video I obtained locally 'Dream Warriors' refused to run the movie but showed another horror drama. I checked the tape with my local video shop and there it played what it was supposed to. Who can imagine my puzzlement and frustration at not being able to explain any of these fantastic occurrences. Visions of a beautiful sun and a river like the ganges flashed on my television and indeed the sun shone brilliantly straight into my flat on occasions as if cradling me or giving me support. I had dreamt that there was a God who loved me and had a purpose for me. His name was Ra but he was an alien. The themes of both sun and moon and their places and functions in our universe were prominent throughout. I badly needed feedback from metaphysicians on what I was experiencing, someone who could give me feedback and enlightenment. But no one was available of such a calibre.

I felt that in dream realities which were another aspect of one's mind, either subconscious, parallel conscious or supra conscious, we can be on different places or worlds or realities. Most of the ones I have encountered are deadly and depleting and it was my intention to get my whole being away from them into more replenishing intelligent and inspirational planes of existence. Dreaming is vital to a knowledge of being, not merely a personal psychology.

I had done much work on the conscious and subconscious mind but in my current state I cannot digress on this. I am not fit to return to this work unless I am healed, balanced and normal. I was angry that my personal work had been raped and seized by these entities, years of hard slog and personal sacrifice using myself as a guinea pig. I had had no protection and felt angry that somehow my feminine gender and lack of social status had been used against me. I know of no other woman in my particular field and have sufficient material collected for four or five books. My book "The Race Odyssey" may never be published for it runs counter to current political ideology. Who determines the course of our political and social evolution? It must be a higher power. How much influence does man have, individually and collectively in the force of this unseen power. These are questions which have preoccupied philosophical and religious thought for millenniums. Destiny versus willed determination, or the power of the subconscious versus the conscious.

My own role seemed to be one of performing one of two possible destinies which had been predetermined for me in the year dot. And I confess to having so many deja vu experiences through the battle with Borts and interchanges with my ancestors, as if I already knew about all this or had done or rehearsed it before. That knowledge alone pleased me, for it almost made me responsible for what was occurring whoever 'me' is. For I began my quest long ago with two questions 'Who and what am I?' and 'What the hell am I supposed to be doing here - what is my task or purpose? ''Know thyself and be thyself' should be branded on our flesh at birth. I haven't got very far in my quest, and almost feel I know less now than I knew before. The very foundations of my life and reality as I knew them have been shaken and shattered. How I would re-assemble or re-emerge was an affair of the Gods. One thing is for sure I reiterate my own inviolability from theft and rape by person, God, entity or spirit and the same right for every other individual being whoever or whatever they may be.

In conclusion my keen observation of other psychotic patients confirms to me that they are under siege - mind or body invasion and in need of altogether different methods of treatment from those they are receiving. They are not to blame except for factors over which they have personal control, like the rest of us. Surely somewhere, somehow, someone will find the breakthrough with intelligent co-operation from all fields of enquiry, not just sectionalised, sterile and cut off.

Chapter seven

In December 1988 I went to a residential Christmas workshop run by Leo Rutherford whom I had met in the summer of that year. He struck me as a genuine and perceptive shaman of the human condition and that which lay beyond it. This session was held at Grimstone Manor in Devon and I was given a lift by a Paul Tinger a Dutchman on the quest. Unfortunately Paul felt he couldn't stay on at Grimstone Manor and left to seek his own space. Leo held a session for expressing anger at those who had oppressed us. I told him I wished to murder God who had let me down. He said that was heavy duty and something he wasn't equipped for. Nevertheless despite the hypnagogic dialogue going on at the back of my mind I found the weekend rewarding and useful. Paul Tinger came to pick me up and take me back to London and again I entered an altered state. Paul was extremely worried and suggested I contact a teacher known as Daskalos in Cyprus who could heal and interpret illness.

I kept all this in mind and at a later stage attempted to contact Dr Styilianos.

However I seemed to improve and by the middle of January 1989 I felt I was in the clear and on the mend. I was aware that some sort of alchemy was taking place, as I was willy nilly taken through moods of youth long forgotten, emotions and memories of times and persons long past. This process took place usually as I lay on my bed. One experience was disturbing and that was a tape in an unknown language which I have since labelled Kryptonian, being played inside my head and causing exceeding pain to my brain and also personal distress. It took me to psychic places which were depleting. The main thrust was my daughter Chantal holding a Halloween rite which was injurious to me hence causing strife between us.

I had agreed with my son Adrian to start up a business agency and I was pleased that I would be able to occupy some of my time arranging the business by telephone. My one and only completed book "The Race Odyssey" (an offshoot from earlier work black or white, the half caste's dilemma) had been rejected by six publishers' doors. The all consuming urgency was towards wholeness, healing and escape from the metapsychosis and a return to normality.

Alas on the 27th January the day before my twin sons' birthday celebrations at Jacquelin's in town which I had promised myself to go with Paul Tinger my brain emitted a familiar explosion and bang, I was plunged into an altered state in minutes, if not seconds. A fellow patient at Chase Farm Hospital has accurately and aptly stated that there is no way to fight a psychosis, you just have to go along with it wherever it takes you. My friend also stated a prayer that the beings and realities encountered on these trips should not be real i.e substantiate into our 'ordinary world. I agree with him for without exception I have encountered only horror in these states. The only exception were the broadcasts that continued to be channelled through my television and radio cassette, and the occasional humour I could muster when Ian Borts kept attempting to materialise, seduce and browbeat me on these hard to define planes. I suppose mediums call it the spirit world, a term I don't like for the spirit means something totally different to me, i.e. fire and goodness. I prefer to distinguish these places forces or realities by the term occult or non-ordinary fields of experience. Carlos Casteneda has useful definitions such as 'heightened awareness' and the vast generic term "the second attention". I call my own simply 'altered state' or a hypnagogic hold' which is conscious but difficult to recall once I return to what medics call reality and I call normality.

Several months elapsed since my recent re-entry into metapsychosis and there is no way that I would give a detailed chronological account; especially as I was told in some way or another that these events constituted an experiment with time and no time. What was the final purpose of the ongoing phenomena in my life I'm not quite sure. Two plots were recalled: the first was the annihilation or mutilation of human beings who were seen by some supreme intelligence as nothing more than spiders crawling on the ground; the second was the takeover of intelligence by workmen - the latter plot sounds fantastic but was plausible when explored. Both designs were horrendously evil in their aim and experience. I must emphasize that in a psychotic state every item takes on a sharp significance, everything is vital to the plot, even the shape of a pin and its placement on the table. I 'was told' always means telepathically; my communications were all telepathic both ways and as intelligible and informative as speech. The major frustration was not having a physical, tangible presence to relate to; the latter only appeared in visions or dreams.

On the 28th January my flat was moved once more, only this time it was in ultimate terror. I went in pitch darkness to nowhere; my cats didn't accompany me and by now their responses were numbed by various drugs, powder like, that wafted through my windows. Presumably the same power or force moved my belongings, continued to pilfer, abstract and steal my clothes, money, cigarettes and much worse my personal papers and letters. Each dematerialisation was instant, silent and totally non detectable. Very valuable correspondence from my friend Bill Webb vanished. I was furious and desperate at not having it returned; these letters to me and mine to him were to form the basis of a book entitled ' A Spiritual Soap Opera' and had much information on The Speakers and their Jonestown effect on those they had contacted.

Anyhow I digress. Outer space was the worst experience to date. I was crying and wailing like a banshee with little chance of anyone hearing me again. My daughter and grandson who lived upstairs vanished from sight or sound. I was alone gazing at an unfamiliar ceiling with the letter R embossed in reverse. This letter had two significances. One was that in playing the God game or master game, which I had believed was the only game to play, I had decided I didn't like the way creation had moulded me and I was determined to re-educate Rita, i.e. God whoever that being might be. I truly felt I could do a better job, and at one stage in the proceedings applied for a post in the Creator's corridors of power. I had been told there were four Lords of Creation and a fifth unknown. My appeals had all been directed to reveal impeccable intelligence, especially as my sacred discs were cracked open and a covenant emerged on the most amazing cosmology. The second significance of R was a woman I had met in Montreal during The Speakers spiritual weekend. She had continued to be in touch with me by sending publicity concerning another trans medium group called Reflections.

The latter was run by Steve and Donna Kinnerborough who had at one stage trained Ian Borts. I never knew why Rita Truba sent me this unwanted information without a personal message, but on my radio cassette I heard a broadcast. A very yuppyish up market voice booming out at me 'Re-educating Rita' you will go mad mad mad! Obviously someone, somewhere had had excellent access to my life, work and thoughts. This was further substantiated by so many television broadcasts which were ironic riders to my written work on politics, race, metaphysics and ontology.

Anyhow in outer space I was petrified. My body was implanted with ice and electricity in order to press bleep buttons for escape from what I was told were Martians, The

Speakers and my bloodline the Inglotts. The latter figured prominently throughout the proceedings as prime initiators of all the plots and rituals. My dead father Tony was around for a lot of the time performing many roles vis a vis my life, both good and bad. The bad part seemed to occur when I lost consciousness, and, on coming to, found that my left hand had been slashed to show I had been sold by my father to the devil. For a long time I have the scar to mark the slash. The same night I saw 'Rosemary's Baby' on the box; the message was clear. Everyone seemed fed up with God and in agreement that he needed to be murdered by Satan. My flat and territory were eventually moved back to a more familiar position, but for days the skies at night and morning were different from what I had grown used to. I'm not an astronomer so will not attempt to describe the heavens. However two states were terrifying; the first was pitch darkness at dawn and the second was the appearance of dawn at three am with birds singing. These phenomena continued for several months together with other stellar movements, satellites winking and one bonafide spaceship, a true flying saucer fairly high in the sky. The evil now centred on beings who loved cruelty and became sexually excited by others' suffering.

It was horrible and I did my utmost to dissolve these realities with the communications I had available; one was the Christ though I never felt his gentleness, only his power and strangely enough his pride. The other figure was a woman I called Freya, or the Ice Queen. Her origins and roles were not easily definable but she helped me through several astral voyages and dialogues with the dead. I saw her in holograms outside my window, and the dead were seen as projected coffins and images in sharp dark outline on my walls. Everything in my flat threw a strange shadow, often a double or treble one, including my body, pretty unnerving actually especially when I saw life size shadows at my front door and felt their threatening enormity.

Between the 28th January and 16th February 1989 I went through several experiences of non-ordinary reality, many were rituals, totally comprehensible and justified at the time of their occurrence, but now ridiculous and unnerving in the cold clime of reason. I met my daughter Chantal and my sister in law Lindsay through this frightening phase and to me they appeared undead, vampires who were totally unaware of their condition, which is not evident when I see them in a normal reality. Much of my information had to do with Ian Borts, The Speakers, my family and the amount of information I was dealing out on the science of being. My father took over much of the proceedings telling me that he was Death itself and very powerful as an invasion or electric force. His design was to unfold my destiny and take pride in a daughter who had so much knowledge in these altered states. It is true that my thoughts in a psychic state are strangely more informative and impactful than in an ordinary state. It seemed that The Speakers wanted to 'borrow' my brain or hold me as a hostage for them to reach another galaxy.

When I listened to their tapes in Montreal they had stated that they were searching the galaxies to find their friends who had vanished, and that they wanted to move from their position where they created all their realities instantly. It is a pity that I destroyed all The Speakers tapes during both my psychoses as I could now play them to experts who might be able to throw more light on these entities. At this point I was unable to proceed further with my tale due to the withdrawal of my life force and my reduction to a zombie like state which lasted for two years. I lived like an embryo throughout that time incapable of performing the simplest task. I now take up the narrative in 1998 to complete my experiences in a psychosis that with only very few intermissions lasted for one year and the subsequent events.

One of the most puzzling experiences were the television broadcasts I was receiving. These were channelled on BBC2 very early in the morning. The title was B.M.T.V which I took to mean British Medical Television. The broadcasts were all in a strange language which I continued to call Kryptonian. The subject matter was medical - medicines, hypodermic needles and operations. The Speakers had declared themselves experts on medical cures and I could only assume that they were exhibiting their expertise on my television.

The other experience which was unnerving was that the Ayatollah Khomeni zoomed in on my reality. He had seized Salmon Rushdie and told me that my work on the Race Odyssey was as powerfully anti-establishment as Rushdie's work on the Satanic Verses. In fact I saw Salman Rushdie twice on television. On one occasion he was looking at splendid looking space beings and on another occasion he was deformed and degraded.

I grew tired of the Khomeni's attentions even though I was told he was an initiate monitoring rebirth. He was torturing me and yet in some strange way it wasn't personal. He informed me that I would have made a good advisor to his government. One night after torture I ordered his death. Imagine my amazement when I saw his assassination broadcast on television the following day. But he then appeared to me as the Holy Man of the East and offered me his personal protection. The problem of teleports continued. One night a man was teleported into my flat. I was petrified and left the flat through the back door. I ran along the North Circular towards Arnos Grove. To my amazement I saw my friend Don Smythe Macaulay walking towards me. I rushed up to him and flung my arms around him telling him we must contact the police to evict the man in my flat. Don didn't speak a word but followed me nervously down the road towards the telephone booth. But when I turned around he had disappeared. It was all an illusion or a question of meeting the person's double. Anyhow I tried to get through to the police without success and was forced to return to my flat where the stranger had disappeared. Then my son Adrian was teleported into the flat. He was whirling like a dervish and said this was the way to reach the cosmos. Whereupon he vanished through the ceiling. My horror was maximal. The next teleport was Leon. He appeared in front of me and told me to go back where I came from, which puzzled me for I didn't know where I came from. He further told me that he was co-operating with my father Tony in an experiment with time and I knew how fastidious my father was about time keeping. I was flabbergasted but in the next instant Leon disappeared. Chantal my daughter then appeared with a friend of mine Evelyn. Chantal said they had better wash the evil off their faces and then Evelyn said "all this belongs to me now". I was astounded but again the two disappeared.

Around the same time I was carried off in the middle of the night to have special lenses inserted in my eyes. I was terrified and the next day went to visit the optician to ask him to remove these lenses, but of course the optician could find no foreign objects in my eyes. Around this time too The Speakers carried me off to the fenced off territory opposite my flat. They showed me a beauty queen performance of deformed women and I laughed. But it seemed because I had been amused by this bizarre display they dumped me in this fallow land and left me to rot.

Ultimately it seemed to be a game of the Gods each one competing to create life. I fell madly in love with each God who presented himself to me but most of all with the Magician who was father and lover rolled into one. He converted the skies, the oceans, and the earth but was ultimately controlled by the unknown fifth Lord of Creation

Chapter eight

From January to July 1989 I was plagued with psychosis, yet I felt there was nothing wrong with me and all I needed was a neurophysiologist to examine my brain. I had a death machine that could perform the most extraordinary tasks. It could convert horror into clouds of glory, and moreover designed my future lives. I saw that my son Adrian was also a victim in generations to come. But the ultimate hold on my machine was held by The Speakers. I had to press the floorboards before the machine became activated. I also had to press my mattress to obtain cigarettes. I could not believe that cigarettes manifested themselves on my bed just by pressing the mattress.

Anyhow I was constantly being tortured and finally in July 1989 I went to casualty at Chase Farm Hospital demanding to see a neurophysiologist. I was promptly admitted to the psychiatric ward much to my disgust. I was sectioned for one month. I was given chorpromazine which got me out of the psychosis but left me for dead. I was discharged in a zombified state. I had a new flat in Lodge Drive, Palmers Green and for the next two years I didn't do an iota of cleaning to it. I lived like a zombie during this time. Though I had made a good friend called Philip Brown during this time who used to visit me every Saturday. He gave me support and reassurance, and does so still this day despite the fact that he is living for most of the year in his native South Africa. I rarely saw my children who could not cope with my illness. During this time I read extensively into psychiatric illness and one book struck me as pre-eminently apposite. It was called "Overcoming Schizophrenia " by W.F.Torrey.
He stated that the illness was purely medical, that psychosis damaged the brain and that a third of schizophrenics committed suicide. Suicide was never far from my

thoughts. A friend of mine Colin Long said that what I had lost was incalculable. I had turned into the opposite of what I used to be. From being an outgoing jovial energetic personality I had become totally withdrawn, humourless and inert individual. Just the thought of going into the garage to get petrol left me distraught. The simplest tasks were difficult. I spent my days at Chase Farm Hospital watching the secretaries dart to and fro - it was life and I had no life. Leo and Mo came to see me from time to time but nothing was enough. I was lonely and internally bereft. I was deeply depressed and can only say that I relate completely to William Styron's "Darkness Visible" in the dynamics of clinical depression.

In 1994 I had my third psychosis. The pain was excruciating. Psychiatrically I had reached an all time low and was admitted into Suffolk Ward Chase Farm in a state of collapse. In the meantime Adrian had been refurbishing my living room with a view to moving in as he could no longer remain in his flat. He did move in July 1991 and the joy I felt was immense that I was no longer alone. I was in hospital at the time with severe depression and was admitted for over three months. On my return home Chantal phoned to tell me that Adrian was hooked on crack cocaine. I was heartbroken. It explained so much of what had been going on in his life. Never daunted I launched on a blitz campaign on clearing up the flat knowing how much Adrian hated dirt. I was helped by a fellow patient Eileen Murphy whose wisdom I respect till this day even though I no longer see her. Adrian and I settled down to domestic life each of us with our own handicaps.

In late 1981 both Adrian and I made journeys abroad. Adrian went to Freetown Sierra Leone to stay with Donald Smythe-Macauley in the hope that medicine men could wean him off his addiction. Alas this was not to be. I personally don't have much confidence in shamans.

75

Though I too was making a journey to meet a man of knowledge Daskalos or Dr Stylianos. I had been told by Paul that he was a miraculous healer. When I arrived in Cyprus and went to stay with a friend, Ian Little in Paphos I contacted Daskalos in Nicosia. His daughter told me that her father was fully booked up till January of next year and couldn't see me. My disappointment knew no bounds. She asked me in the meantime to write a letter explaining my symptoms and enclosing a photograph, which I did but never received an answer. I cut my stay in Paphos short as I was suffering from severe panic attacks and returned to London after a week.

I then had to watch my son destroy himself on crack. We had several altercations some of them violent. Adrian complained about how my mental illness placed a strain on him, and I complained about the financial hardship that his habit placed on our finances. Despite our conflicts we both became very co-dependant and I reached a stage where I could not envisage life without Adrian supporting me emotionally.

During this period I had developed a close relationship with my psychiatrist Dr Michael Bowman. He saw me once a week for therapy. Though strictly speaking these were not therapeutic sessions but rather intervals where I could exercise what was left of my intellectual powers on someone equally intellectual. I showed off my knowledge of mental illness until Dr Bowman acknowledged that I knew as much about it as he did. At one stage he asked my opinion on a patient on the ward admitting he was wrong in doing this. Alas our relationship deteriorated as I became more and more emotionally distressed. Dr Bowman seemed unable to carry my general hysteria and suddenly announced that I was not at all mentally ill. Apparently I was suffering from a personality disorder, a narcissistic personality, and second he wouldn't see me anymore until I took a job as a barmaid in a pub. I was shocked and horrified and proceeded to write Dr Bowman several letters of explanation and protest. He said he found my letters interesting but sent back a batch to me after I'd arrived drunk at his office and asked him if he didn't want to learn more about mental illness. I was specifically referring to the psychic aspect of the illness particularly possession in which he said he didn't believe. I asked for a second opinion from the Charing Cross Hospital which Dr Bowman tried to block. I had to appeal to my member of parliament Michael Portillo to get the referral. After this I was admitted to the Charing Cross Hospital on three or four occasions. The nursing care there was better than at Chase Farm but the environment was not as congenial. Professor Hirsh at the Charing Cross Hospital diagnosed me as a manic depressive with neurotic problems. I disagree with his diagnosis. For practical reasons I could no longer receive treatment from the Charing Cross Hospital which was far out of my catchment area so I had to return to Chase Farm. But my treatment was eventually handed over to Dr Mary Cody, a pleasant but somewhat ineffectual psychiatrist.

In early 1993 I stopped taking drugs for my illness and by the middle of the year my depression lifted and my emotions returned. Together with them came an increasing desire to seek a cure for my mental problems. I reached some sort of crisis in July 1993 and was admitted to Chase Farm Hospital. I experienced agony in my solar plexus and then a great feeling of anguish as my mind returned in an avalanche of new epistemology (the study of the science of knowledge). At the same time my emotions reached new heights - anger at my children and the way they had treated me, and generally anger with the world. I was discharged after about three weeks and returned home where I gave Adrian a stupendous dressing down for his behaviour. He maintained to be suicidal after my onslaught but we somehow recovered an equilibrium for living.

I continued to experience torture through my solar plexus and could only presume that space beings were doing this to me. My emotions hit the roof and I became angry at everything and everyone including New Age teaching, Christianity, the middle classes and anything else I could think of. I used to get up very early in the morning and spend the day putting down all my thoughts on paper to send to Philip Brown in South Africa. My outpourings constituted a book and in the meantime I was in agony with the torture.

I was told that all my psychoses had been set up by the higher selves. I don't like using the term lower self for that is where creativity stems. The pettiness and appetites of the lower self can be injurious but maybe not so disastrous as those of pride and arrogance that proceed from the realms of ideas and life purpose. Nazi Germany is a classic example. It wasn't the lower self that was responsible for the holocaust. None of what happened was for sex or money or petty interests. It was a vision of supremacy that set these actions in motion. As St Paul says our battle is not with flesh and blood but with the principalities and powers that surround this dark planet and evil in the spiritual and heavenly realms. Both the Christ and St.Paul exalt love, the Buddha exalts compassion. I relate more to compassion than to Christian love. I have a distinct instinct that the kind of love that is written in the Xtian context actually doesn't exist in this dimension. The law of survival and self preservation is all too powerful. Maybe it's an ideal but I've know of no one capable of the selflessness expounded in Christian and its allied metaphysical literature. I was not able to love my own son in Christian terms so I have no chance of loving a stranger in this way.

I spent many days in bed with the torture going through my

solar plexus. I was shown in a dream state that one of my four invisible bodies had been seized by The Speakers and their surgeons in outer space. In the same dream state I tried to seize the body back but failed, the work was abandoned.

It was in early 1984 that I was re-reading a diary I had kept in Montreal 1980. I had recorded a dream that a spirit or entity had entered the attic. If alien it would be friendly, if non-alien unfriendly. In either case it had to be captured or faced and I was afraid. This made me more convinced that I was possessed by a spirit. I interpreted the attic as my mind. In fact I made a return visit to the exorcist but felt worse after his exorcism. Frankly it is only cowardice that has kept me alive for I've experienced many kinds of hell and if I had been brave enough I would have thrown myself under a train or put a knife through myself.

During 1993 and early 1994 when my mind and emotions had returned I would have days when I seemed to function fairly normally, then others when I could barely move from the bed, and when I was in a poor emotional state I had trouble sleeping. I also had hypnogogic visions.

I remember thinking once a psychotic always a psychotic, and I did not know what to believe or think anymore. On some days I functioned with intellectual clarity and then on other days this vanished. One patient at Chase Farm Eileen Murphy said ' your God could not stand it any more - he left'. I did say during psychosis - let the spirit go free - I send it into " the bank of the spirit of man". I could never quite understand what the soul was and at one stage said I did not need one - it could be distributed among those who did. Prior to all of this I had never considered myself a candidate for madness. I was highly logical and analytical. The only clue has been the traumatic dreams I've had since childhood - frightening, bizarre with little relationship to anything I have known. So maybe there is latent madness in the unconscious connected to the spiritual self or the monadic structure. In mental illness I have experienced the removal of most of my subconscious banks. An absence of one's mind is inconceivable to a mentally well person. In real terms it means that there is no more thinking flow or internal feeding between conscious and subconscious. It is internal starvation leading to a zombified state needing ongoing external stimulation to keep on existing. Contemporary psychiatry with its pre-eminent emphasis on hit and miss chemotherapy and ancillary counselling or psychological therapy is inadequate to heal these illnesses. The hospitals provide at best a sanctuary, attention (i.e. a form of love) and fellow travellers all of which may catalyse an internal healing process from an unknown place in the psyche.

Chapter nine

Christmas 1993 was a deep crisis point for me and Adrian. Both of us had undergone great instability, mood changes, conflicts and reconciliations. Adrian was deeply depressed and still in the grip of his crack habit. My fear was that he would die. At times he threatened to leave me and this made me frightened and insecure. I couldn't cope on my own. Sometimes I threatened to throw him out when I found his behaviour too confrontational either in attitude or actions or in the individuals he invited into the home. Adrian found my hospital admissions painful and stressful. And I similarly found his anti-social behaviour and the financial strain in obtaining his drugs also stressful. Yet we still remained co-dependent

In August 1993 my other son Leon went to consult the medicine man in Freetown, Sierra Leone to ask for shamanistic help in all our predicaments. He, Pa Salia said that an evil spirit had emerged when their father died in 1967 and had especially affected me and Adrian. The reason he gave was that Adrian and I were not mentally as strong as Leon. I rejected this explanation partially. Adrian and I were emotionally more vulnerable than Leon. However my own seeing in an altered state had shown me that Adrian and I had been chosen for crucifixion because our spines were the strongest and therefore able to withstand the onslaught. Leon at school once had a spinal problem. The entire concept of one's spine in the scheme of things barely crops up in books. It is the seat of all three nervous systems and all the chakras. These are linked to all the layers of the subconscious mind and their connections with the universe and the cosmos i.e. the unknown. My own etheric spine was smashed in psychosis and then repaired and then abstracted in its totality by the demiurge
Saturn who was handing it to my occult opponent Ian Borts.

At the end of 1993 I had become so ill, distressed and terrified that I asked to be admitted to the Charing Cross Hospital. There I told staff what was happening to me. Obviously they did not agree with me but pronounced that I was gravely mentally ill. I was given psychotropic drugs and experienced two grave internal seizures which were even more painful than my illness. My blood pressure rose alarmingly - I ceased to function and wanted instant suicide. I recovered but then had to refuse the drugs. Moreover I did not feel comfortable with most of the other patients. This was unusual as over the years I have got on pretty well with other mentally ill people and have received much support and encouragement from many of them. This time I found no one I could relate to and was disturbed by some who were intrusive, abusive or violent. I did meet one young black girl who said she knew what was happening to me as it was happening to her. It was driving her mad and she was fighting it. She agreed that the doctors would not believe us. I also met another attractive woman, very upper middle class who felt comfortable with her psychic experiences, i.e. protected and like myself was addicted to pain killers. I also felt I needed barbiturates to tide me over. However the current medical climate is very anti barbiturates and Professor Hirsh was quite scathing over what he called my addiction to barbiturates. I discharged myself before I was sectioned.

I returned home to Adrian who was supportive and sympathetic. I also continued to see Leo Rutherford who gave me encouragement and support. My psychic centres had re-opened and I begun to have hypnageagic visions. I saw Adrian standing with arms outstretched, his veins strangely prominent and he had a knife ready to slash them. The I saw him shouting at me aggressively and then suddenly collapsing into tears. The first vision corresponded to his intermittent threats of suicide in recent months. The second vision showed " when you feel pain you inflict pain". I realised how much emotional pain Adrian still felt. I also pondered on how often aggression is a cover up for suppressed pain. Personally I've understood how an intolerably high level of frustration can lead to berserk reactions like crashing one's car or indiscriminate killing. I have felt like doing these things and controlled myself, perhaps through prudence i.e.the fear of the result of such actions.

Back to my missing body. I had a very brief glimpse that it was in a room and in an esoteric book I read that I had four bodies. I also dreamt of the card Justice in the tarot pack - not an easy card but one of difficulties and Karmic justice. The following morning I questioned my deck and the card Justice turned up. Gog and Magog briefly appeared as they did in 1932 in my first drug mind expansion. Philip told me these were not very beneficial figures and manifested at the end of the world. I was then told to beware of the geminian betrayal. I once jokingly wrote that one twin had gone home she could not stand it anymore. I have gemini rising in my birth chart. Leane a healer Rosicrucian friend told me that Cheiron the healer is in Gemini in my chart. I also had a highly lucid dream. Leo was sitting on my bed telling me to put my finances in order. He had in his hands an unidentified magazine in which I was interested. However I was unable to get very much information from Leo on the magazine. But I glanced inside the magazine and Howard Charing was advertised as a healer of mental illness. Leo then pointed to Saturn in Aquarius in my birth chart saying it meant I would not get what I wanted. This message made me feel disappointed.

I had another lucid dream where Adewole John a former lover was threatening to beat me up and finish me off. About ten unknown men were present. I turned to each one for help but to my shock and fear they all retreated got into a lift and descended out of sight. Adewole then said he wasn't going to carry out his threat anyway and said "everyone wants Bianca Benjamin". This dream illustrates that my animus is weak and doesn't support me when the chips are down.

During my last admission to the Charing Cross Hospital I followed Howard's exercise of stating that I take two more steps into the light. He had told me that I feared the light. Imagine my horror when as I was walking along the corridor my mind was removed. I was terrified and told the staff (unbelieving I'm sure). How was all this being done invisibly. I went into further darkness and despair. I had during this period experienced no forces or presences surrounding me. Though once I felt pressure beside me on the bed. The cats no longer slept on my bed. Amber who was demonised in psychosis two developed a spinal infection and later had to be put down. Adrian too became physically very ill though giving me a lot of support at this time.

After my discharge I had a fleeting dream telling me I had always been lucky and I would be lucky again. I consulted the tarot and got the Hierophant the Speaker card. They had my missing body. I also did a runic spread giving me the past as flow of emotions, the outcome standstill, and the conclusion constraint. The future held wholeness and healing. Throughout the whole period between the summer of 1993 and 1994 I experienced daily and sometimes hourly uncertainties and instabilities.

Carlos Castaneda during this time had published a further book "The Art of Dreaming". I found it a total disappointment. It did not inspire or ring bells. Just a few messages; first, to live without the nagual the spirit is worse than death. Then that the energy of inorganic beings sizzles while ours wavers. I had dreamt that I was preparing food for Adrian in a Pyrex dish on the worktop and not on the stove. The food was sizzling hot and burning. I was dismayed, trying to stop it. I could not and the food splattered over the work top and to my horror shrank - what would Adrian eat? Since the unknown zoomed in on me again Adrian no longer wanted me to cook for him. His reason was that I had burned the food and he no longer liked my cooking.

Leo had urged me to read the "Art of Dreaming" purely for its information on inorganic beings who feed on our energy and give us knowledge in return. He felt that The Speakers may have fallen into this category.

During this period I received an edition of "Human Potential" edited and produced by Aaron Gersh who had been sending me free copies for years. But none had moved me as his edition on compassion. It was jam packed with re-echoed long forgotten truths and I understood it from cover to cover. Basically it stated the law of compassion overrides all other laws. Moreover it stated that the premise that we alone create our own suffering is highly dangerous. Which brings me back to The Speakers who stated that we alone create everything in our world. But which 'I' creates? In psychosis I saw that the whole drama had been set up by the higher selves.

In early 1994 I had another hypnologic vision of the rune of initiation both the right and the wrong way around. I had picked this rune some years earlier as my task in this life. It is the rune of mystery and of the Phoenix Rising from the ashes to new life. A very active Rosicrucian called Okon had come to visit me and stated that I was not mentally ill at all but initiating. Yet I maintain that for a long time I had been suffering from spiritual AIDS. Maybe my monad was sick and bankrupt. I have dreamt that I have problems in the subconscious mind.

I realised at one stage that I of myself could do nothing. My physical vehicle is just a shell but one that undergoes horrendous suffering. Of myself there is nothing to be done. The source of the ability to feed is numinous and invisible.

As one priest I met in Malta said - without God i.e. the spirit, there is no love; no hate either I should imagine.

One day in May 1994 while I was writing my epistle to Philip I suddenly entered my third major psychosis. As usual The Speakers zoomed in and my fingers were implemented for purposes of communication. We largely discussed Adrian to begin with. But then my body was charged with fire and electricity and I told them I hated them. They said they hated me too. Within a short period I was being strangled internally, the pain was horrendous and the fear of choking to death. I telephoned both my mother and Leo to come and help me but only Leo turned up. He brought some Bach remedies to help me through and gave me much encouragement in my struggle.

I prostrated myself on the floor begging The Speakers to let me go. I said I would worship them if only they stopped strangling me. My daughter Chantal took me to my G.P who issued a letter to Chase Farm Hospital to admit me. I was admitted but by this time I was convinced that my body carried time bombs and atomic warfare. I asked on admission for an X Ray to see what devices were in my body. Obviously I was ignored. I ran away from hospital quite quickly but Adrian could not cope with me in that state and called on Leon's help. Leon had me sectioned and my car keys were taken away.

I saw that the world was dead, the trees were hollow and we were in another reality. All the galaxies had collapsed and there was barely any exit into space. Carlos Castaneda's teacher Don Juan manifested and said he could not travel into the unknown for all the worlds had collapsed.

He also demonstrated the power of silence in which there was perfect peace.

The main thrust of this psychosis was sexual. I was injected with overwhelming sexual feeling and saw that no place in existence could resist the power of sex. The spiritual realms were not exempt and every being succumbed to this sexual impulse. In the meantime I was sequestered in Chase Farm Hospital.

But suddenly I was overcome by a sensation resembling an internal earthquake and I collapsed on the floor. This collapse occurred at regular intervals over a period of months. The feeling of discomfort and disorientation was so intense that it made me feel suicidal. At one stage I ran a bath in order to drown myself but the instinct of self preservation forced me to rise to the surface.

By November 1994 I was considered well enough to be discharged from hospital. Adrian had by this time met an Italian educated German girl Susanne with whom he was planning to live. I dreaded him moving out of the flat. I could not bear to be alone and this psychosis like the previous two left me totally empty and helpless. In any event Adrian did move out in April 1995 and after two weeks I took a massive overdose of medicines which left me unconscious for a couple of days but I came to in hospital with a great feeling of disappointment. By August 1995 Adrian and Susanne had split up largely due to Adrian's drug habit and he moved back in with me. But all was far from well. Adrian was deteriorating mentally, emotionally and psychologically. He admitted himself briefly to a rehabilitation centre in Islington but discharged himself. He threatened suicide but part of me refused to believe that he would actually go through with this.

But I was proved wrong. On the 19th September 1995 he went to Kings Cross and obtained heroin. On the morning of the 20th September I found him lying on the floor, he was dead. I was devastated, that which I feared had come upon me. I am still not reconciled to his death. I was confronted with the problem of evil and its origins. I was taken to a man who embodied evil. He spoke in a dead pan voice which was filled with utter boredom. He represented the principalities of evil that surround this planet. I told him I felt sorry for him and my pity caused him to let me go. Though during the entire interchange I was petrified. Later I was told that evil had originated with the abominable snowman, the yeti and I became ice cold during this revelation.

I was shown much mutilation both of humans and animals. Many of them had been genetically engineered and the experiment had gone drastically wrong. I called in the good forces to clear up the mess. As usual in my psychosis there was a period of laughter and this occurred when I was broadcasting to the astral planes. The antics that The Speakers employed to invade ones privacy. I was adamant that they should not be let in under any circumstances. I made fun of them instead of being afraid and this provided me with much humour.

There was an additional theme that revolved around initiates. It seemed that many souls wanted to initiate. In my own nomadic structure I had Noel Coward bidding for initiation and he comforted me and kept me company throughout much of my psychosis. The theory of reincarnation wasn't made to seem that simple. In my understanding at the time of my altered state it seemed as if one monad sent forth several separate beings into the world who retained their individuality but were bonded by the single monad.

Throughout this psychosis I saw myself as a multiplicity. There was no single 'I'. I had one part of me that had been trapped in the astral plane with Adrian alone in a mental hospital. Another part was light and airy and humorous. Another part of me was in space with an entire space family. I was told that I would find Adrian dead in his room and I panicked. There were further dynamics revolving around Jesus Christ. He was an impostor and I asked that all prayers directed to him should be rerouted to me as I was world saviour.

Most stories have a happy ending. This one does not. I live alone and find the simplest tasks complicated. I have little motivation and am dead within. I suffer from extreme loneliness both internal and external. Most of my friends have withdrawn their attention. I spend some of my time looking after my grandchildren which I find very rewarding. I cannot cry and I cannot laugh, my emotions are deadened. But on the plus side my agoraphobia has almost cleared up and I no longer suffer from crippling panic attacks. I am thankful for the few friends I still have and for the love and support of my two remaining children Chantal and Leon. I would give anything to find a cure for mental illness which is the most crippling of illnesses. But my knowledge of physiology is almost non-existent. I acknowledge Leo Rutherford's crucial role in supporting me throughout these years. It has been suggested to me that I should reduce my medication in order to regain my feelings, but it has also been suggested that I adhere strictly to my medication in order to avoid another psychosis. At present I cannot make up my mind which course to follow. I acknowledge the help and support I have received from other mentally ill people. I am no longer suicidal but the quality of my life leaves much to be desired. I have no belief system and see God as Castaneda's Eagle black and white from whom all emanations flow. This is my story.

Epilogue

The foregoing is a tale about madness which, as they say, is only funny in the late night show. There is the bizarre and extravagance that occurs when entering altered states of perception which psychiatrists call psychoses. Then there is the quite insidious insanity that accompanies clinical depression. There is also the ongoing crippling agony of panic attacks emanating from either the heart region or the solar plexus.

William Styron the author of 'Sophie's Choice' became clinically depressed late in life and at the height of his career. In his concise and powerful book 'Darkness Visible' he describes deep depression as a life threatening illness equally as serious as cancer or diabetes. Desire for suicide is constantly present and one is reduced to a zombie like state. Styron eventually came through this illness after being admitted to a psychiatric clinic.

Schizophrenia has a bad press largely because a small minority are violent and uncontrollable. The majority tend to be withdrawn like myself. Manic depression has more status as it has afflicted many creative personalities throughout time.

I have survived many potential fatal illnesses such as meningitis, cancer, deep vein thrombosis and one anaphylactic shock. There is a sense in which I have survived mental illness. I have had no psychotic episodes for over seven years nor experienced clinical depression for six years. The panic attacks have also ceased. Yet I feel neither anguish nor joy. I cannot laugh wholeheartedly nor can I except on rare occasions cry. I feel alienated and withdrawn in the company of normally functioning human beings.

What is the function of psychiatric hospitals from the viewpoint of the mentally ill. At best the wards provide asylum from an impossibly demanding and frightening outside world. But despite the strides that have been made in the profession over time the care is by and large barbaric. There is virtually no emotional support and staff have become hardened to our suffering. Psychiatrists' main function is to prescribe medication or electro convulsive therapy. They ask stupid questions such as what did you have for breakfast; what day is it; how are you getting on with your brother; count backwards from a hundred to one. I was asked if I whish to harm myself, My reply was why should I wish to harm myself, I want to kill myself.

Consultants do not truly know the cause of schizophrenia nor is there any conclusive cure. I have intuited that there are seven broad causes of mental illness. These are genetic, neuropsychological, psychological, emotional, psychic, spiritual and environmental. Two or more causes may predominate in any individual. In my own case there is no history of mental illness in my family. My causes were emotional psychic, spiritual and environmental. I've had problems with remaining emotionally stable most of my adult life. I have been addicted to tobacco for fifty years and to alcohol for thirty five. Opening my psychic centres was a mistake and I had written in my notes that I was suffering from spiritual AIDS. My environment was poor and isolated with the only person giving me support, my son Leon.

The mentally ill are only too often discharged before they are ready to cope on their own outside. They need twenty four hour support. The community have nothing in common with the mentally ill where they are largely ignored or treated as outcasts. Normally functioning people have little sympathy for those who are mentally afflicted. The latter are regarded as malingering or self indulgent. The mentally ill also have nothing in common with the community and generally speaking socialise with their own kind. Usually there is a three times weekly visit from a community nurse and if one is lucky a visit from a social worker. However this is minimal support and usually a session with one's psychiatrist is on a three monthly basis. The main support both on the ward and on the outside comes from fellow sufferers who understand what it is all about. They do not offer stupid advice like the one given to my by two male nurses that what I needed was some good sex. They, knowing my West African connections proposed that I approach a West Indian stud on one of the wards.

My friend and long standing supporter Leo Rutherford who is a New Age Shaman has advised that my flattened emotions are a result of the psychotropic medication I take. New Age teachings have contributed much to the body of esoteric knowledge. There are also many groups and individuals who assist in self development. However the movement has also attracted many charlatans who use gimmicks to extract money from clients. It has also produced power hungry gurus whose chief motive is to possess the minds of their followers and also make megabucks.

While studying metaphysics I paid frequent visits to the College of Psychic studies. I consulted several mediums who were all without exception entirely wrong about my future. I now believe that the future cannot be foretold. I myself developed an expertise in reading the tarot cards but did not pretend to know the future only current trends in the life. I also practised ritual magic on a regular basis. I now realise that it can be highly dangerous to embark on occult and psychic practices alone without the guidance of a reputable expert. There are all sorts of nasty demons and entities that can be evoked from alternative realities. Since my mental illness I have given up these disciplines.

During these years of mental stress I have received support from various sources. MIND in Barnet were extremely helpful, Sue Townes and Bill Ambler were always there to listen. Unfortunately they both left after my second psychosis. My church was always there to provide visits and comfort. Father Robin Whitney in addition gave much financial aid when my son Adrian was living with me. All our money went on crack cocaine. Some friends also stood by me but on the whole they were people I had met while mentally ill. There was Philip Brown, Leo Rutherford and Colin Long. The latter had known me prior to my collapse and has stated that what I have lost is incalculable. I used to have a vibrant charismatic and vital personality together with a brilliant mind. Now all that has gone and the realm of ideas and concepts is closed to me. I am unable to collate my notes on ontology and epistemology into books.

Which all brings me to the existence of an all good knowing and loving god. Despite my Catholic convent upbringing I spent most of my adult life as an agnostic. However in Montreal 1980 I turned to a Christian god and his son Jesus Christ. I prayed constantly but my prayers were never answered. I no longer believe in this god nor that Christ was god incarnate. Like the Gnostics I affirm that this planet is governed by demiurges. I am seduced by Carlos Castaneda's Eagle (Though Eagle is only a manner of speaking) black and white from whom all emanations flow. As it says in the Old Testament 'I the Lord send it all the good and the bad'.

In the years prior to my last psychosis I tried everything and went everywhere to cure my maladies. I took the Bach remedies, St John's Wart and engaged in Buddhist chanting. I frequented counsellors, psychotherapists, private psychiatrists, healers, psychics and shamans. All to no avail. As mentioned in the text I even travelled with great difficulty to Cyprus to consult Dr. Stylianos commonly called simply Daskalos for miraculous healing of both physical and mental illness. I was unable to see him as he was booked up for months in advance. My ongoing panic attacks caused me to cut my visit short. All was to no avail. From nineteen ninety five I have accepted that there is no known cure for schizophrenia.

Prior to my illness I had agonised on the concept of choice in one's life. As far as I could see I had never really had any real choice in my life. Those imprisoning genes and the environment in which they are plunged are starred at birth and go only in the direction they know how. I am a fatalist and believe like Castaneda that there are powers that guide all living things. He also asserts that the course of a warrior's destiny is unalterable. He can weep buckets on his path but all his tears will not alter his destiny one breadth of an inch. He has only one choice, he can face it as a warrior or as a nincompoop.

Just a postscript. Just before his death Ian Borts in collaboration with Bill Webb had a booked entitled "The Healer" accepted by Simon and Shuster for publication. He was hailed as the Modern Edgar Cayce of our time and was to make a seven city tour of the United States. I told him during our battle that he would make the tour in his coffin. Ian Borts died before he could make the trip and Bill Webb died riddled with cancer in Australia in ninety one. So much for the healer.

I shall end with a quotation from Scott Peck's inimitable book "The Road Less Travelled", "In chronic mental illness there is no growth and the human spirit shrivels".

POSTSCRIPT

I wrote this book early in the year 2000, while I was semi zombified and in a state of ongoing low-grade depression.

Towards the end of summer my depression became severe and I considered cancelling my projected trip to Malta after a seventeen-year absence. I was to make the journey with Leon and his family. However, both friends and relatives persuaded me to go ahead with the holiday and I did so.

On arrival in Gozo, where we had rented a farmhouse, my depression lifted. However, I found that I could make no meaningful connection with my cousins and old friends. I was struck dumb and felt totally alienated. I just kept repeating that I was suffering from schizophrenia. There was one exception, Tara Kilbride Jones, who was and is a manic-depressive. We spent two hours exchanging our experiences.

On my return to London life continued in its customary boredom, loneliness and phases of depression. In late 2003 I once again became fatally ill. My spine collapsed, my internal organs all failed, and I slipped into a coma. I had a tracheotomy and was put on a life support machine in the intensive care unit of Chase Farm hospital. The medical staff told my children that there was little hope that I would pull through.

However, once again I escaped the grim reaper. I regained consciousness and for many weeks I was fed, watered and medicated via drips. I was an inpatient for three months, but on discharge found I could not walk. I used a wheelchair for two months. However, I was determined to become mobile and eventually was able to go short distances with a stick. Now I can walk without aid for medium lengths.

The salient and most important factor in this dicing with death was that my mind set had changed. My consciousness had expanded and parts of my subconscious mind had returned. I was flooded with ideas and could now interact with normal people. Leo was delighted at the change and gave me a lot of encouragement. I am now working on another booked unrelated to mental illness. Its title is 'Black or White, The Half Caste's Dilemma'.

However, my recovery is still only partial, as my etheric body is still imprisoned by the Speakers. I recently consulted a Dr Alan Sanderson, who appeared in an article on exorcism in The Daily Mail. He was cited as a psychiatrist who had success with what he called spirit release. However, Alan said that recovering this body was a difficult task. He relaxed me and guided me to this body. Although this was not very successful as I only have psychic ability while I dream. I am undecided as to whether I shall return to him for further sessions.

Muriel Henderson has told me there is an American woman, Caroline Myss, who can locate the subtle bodies; she works with brain surgeons and can tell what is wrong with their patients. She has written 'Anatomy of the Spirit' and 'Sacred Contracts'. Leo Rutherford has met her in the UK, and if she makes another journey here he will let me know. I feel she could help me, as I do still have presences around me. I know this through my cats, who are highly aware of them.

If I were to write 'Madness at Midnight' now, it would be differently constructed. However, it must stand as a statement in its original form.

The essential point I wanted to emerge from my book has not been clear in the manuscript due to my lack of cohesive thought in the year 2000. I am firmly convinced, as the ancients were, that the majority of mentally ill people are possessed. This possession can be spirits benign or malevolent, demons, entities from other universes or discarnate humans. The voices that schizophrenics hear are not coming from inside their heads but from the possessing entity.

The causes of possession are not always clear. They could be genetic as in the sins of the fathers visiting on the children. There is also karmic element, a residue action from past lives. However I feel that the main trigger is severe emotional or physical trauma, which weakens the immune system and allows an alien force to enter the human being. Excessive use of illicit drugs or alcohol can also prove a breeding ground to those who are susceptible. The current scientific attitude to mental illness only focuses on the physiological and psychological aspects of the disease. The psychic and spiritual factors are ignored, no progress will be made in a cure until attitudes and treatment change. These include alternative healing . In extreme cases exorcism or spirit release is needed. Other methods include cleansing the aura, the use of Reiki or Tai chi, acupuncture, herbal remedies and the giving of much love and attention on a one to one bias. As a matter of interest Dr Bowman told me that autopsies preformed on dead mentally ill individuals showed no physiological abnormalities. This is not to deny the value of medication in controlling symptoms.

In my own case I was initially possessed following intense physical and emotional trauma in Montréal in 1980. I nearly lost my life, later my occult involvement with Ian Borts and the speakers compounded the possession. after my second major psychosis I dreamt that I had been submitted to horrific magic, spiral in nature. I also saw that there was an evil genie in my flat. Involvement with the occult can at times lead to the entry of evil entities into the body and mind.

It is my desire to persuade contemporary psychiatry to adopt a more inclusive and holistic approach to this painful illness. They need to accept that the paranormal does exist.